Murder, Magic, and Medicine

Murder, Magic, and Medicine

John Mann

Oxford ◇ New York ◇ Tokyo
OXFORD UNIVERSITY PRESS
1992

Oxford University Press, Walton Street, Oxford OX2 6DP
Oxford   New York   Toronto
Delhi   Bombay   Calcutta   Madras   Karachi
Kuala Lumpur   Singapore   Hong Kong   Tokyo
Nairobi   Dar es Salaam   Cape Town
Melbourne   Auckland   Madrid
and associated companies in
Berlin   Ibadan

Oxford is a trade mark of Oxford University Press

Published in the United States
by Oxford University Press Inc., New York

A catalogue record for this book is available from the British Library

Library of Congress Cataloging in Publication Data
Mann, J.
Murder, magic and medicine / John Mann.
Includes bibliographical references and index.
1. Pharmacology—history.   2. Folk medicine.   I. Title.
RM300.M1845   1992   615'.1'09—dc20   92–7458

ISBN 0–19–855561–X

Set by
Footnote Graphics, Warminster, Wilts

Printed in Great Britain by
St. Edmundsbury Press, Bury St. Edmunds, Suffolk

Preface

When we visit the doctor we usually want a drug to treat our ailments. We rarely give any thought to the way in which the drug was discovered. More often than not it will have evolved in some way from a folk medicine or from some other natural product. This book seeks to reveal the links between the folk use of plant and animal extracts and their modern use as drugs. No previous knowledge of science or medicine is assumed, and the few chemical structures which are included simply show how the shapes of drug molecules influence their biological activities.

As with any book, numerous people have helped in its production. I am particularly grateful to the following: James Crabbe who helped to ensure that the chemical structures are informative rather than daunting; Dr Jeffrey Aronson who provided invaluable pharmacological (and grammatical!) advice; William Schupbach who revealed to me the marvellous store of photographs in the Wellcome Institute for the History of Medicine; my editor at the Press who masterminded the whole operation with enthusiasm and efficiency; and my wife Rosemary, for her usual forebearance and support.

Finally, I should like to dedicate this book to the memory of my father, who had no formal education beyond the age of thirteen, but developed a passion for all things scientific, and ensured that I received the education that he had been denied.

July 1992   J.M.

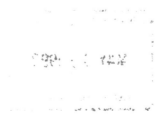

Contents

Introduction

◇

Double, double toil and trouble;
Fire burn and cauldron bubble.
Fillet of a fenny snake,
In the cauldron boil and bake;
Eye of newt, and toe of frog,
Wool of bat, and tongue of dog,
Adder's fork, and blind-worm's sting,
Lizard's leg, and howlet's wing,
For a charm of powerful trouble,
Like a hell-broth boil and bubble.
Double, double toil and trouble;
Fire burn and cauldron bubble.
Scale of dragon, tooth of wolf,
Witches' mummy, maw and gulf
Of the ravin'd salt-sea shark,
Root of hemlock digg'd i' the dark,
Liver of blaspheming Jew,
Gall of goat, and slips of yew
Sliver'd in the moon's eclipse,
Nose of Turk, and Tartar's lips,
Finger of birth-strangled babe
Ditch-deliver'd by a drab,

Introduction

Make the gruel thick and slab:
Add thereto a tiger's chaudron,
For the ingredients of our cauldron.
Double, double toil and trouble;
Fire burn and cauldron bubble.
Cool it with a baboon's blood,
Then the charm is firm and good.

Macbeth, IV, i

This is probably the best known potion in the English language; but did it work? Many of the ingredients, like parts of bats, wolves, Jews, Turks, and unchristened babies, were associated with magic or were simply non-Christian, but a firm belief in such hocus-pocus was not enough to ensure that 'finger of birth-strangled babe' or 'Tartar's lips' proved efficacious. The potency lay with the toxic parts of plants and reptiles, like 'slips of yew', 'root of hemlock', and 'lizard's leg'; and, although the 'eye of newt' and 'toe of frog' are products of Shakespeare's vivid imagination, there is no doubt that his witches had cooked up a thoroughly poisonous brew.

Of course, toxic plant and animal products were widely used long before Shakespeare's time. Primitive man undoubtedly identified edible and poisonous plants and animals by a process of trial and error, and then went on to exploit the toxic materials for executions, euthanasia, murder, and most importantly for hunting.

Despite the abundance of these poisons and their utility to the hunters, food was none the less often in short supply, and most cultures discovered plants which contained substances that would alleviate their misery by providing appetite suppressants, stimulants, and psychedelics. Opium, for example, has been used for at least 5000 years and cocaine for at least 2000 years.

In most prosperous or settled communities, there was time for experimentation, and certain members of the tribe became expert in the selection and use of plant extracts for magic and 'communication with the gods'. These same 'medicine men' recognized the medicinal value of these and other plants, and used them for the benefit of the community and for their own advancement. Take, for example, the ancient Egyptian remedy for a colicky child: 'poppy pods and fly dirt'. The identity of the latter ingredient is not clear, but if the poppy pods were in reality seed capsules from the opium poppy, the major constituent, morphine, would certainly have had a soothing effect on the child's gastrointestinal tract.

Human cultures have, it seems, always had a near fanatical interest in their digestive organs, and in particular a preoccupation with bowel function. In seventeenth century England bimonthly purging was thought to be essential for good health; but long before this the Emperor Shen Nung was recommending the use of rhubarb in his pharmacopoeia (*c.* 2700 BC). The Ebers papyrus (*c.* 1550 BC), found near Luxor in Egypt, also includes rhubarb, along with various species of aloes, castor oil, and senna. The latter was at one time so highly prized that it was reserved for the aristocracy and was known as 'guardian of the royal bowel movement'. The lower castes had to make do with castor oil mixed with beer, and they consumed this brew at least three times a month.

Today we do not usually have the fanatical preoccupation with our bowels that tormented our forebears (though sales of laxatives are still very considerable), but the remedies that we buy are often the same as those which were prescribed 5000 years ago. The same can be said for many of the medicines that we use, and the aim of this book is to demonstrate how at least some of the substances used for murder, magic, and folk medicine have been successfully transformed into clinically acceptable drugs.

Since these plant and animal products exert their effects through the changes that they produce in the physiological and biochemical systems of our bodies, the remainder of this introduction is devoted to the essentials of pharmacology for those not familiar with the subject. Important chemical structures are presented in a form that will allow the reader to obtain an impression of their shape, without having to appreciate the complexity of the chemical bonding which determines these shapes.

Some basic pharmacology

The first primitive mammals appeared on the planet some 200 million years ago, and the human form is one outcome of numerous subsequent evolutionary changes. New chemical constituents and biochemical processes were the ultimate products of these changes, and as a result each member of the species *Homo sapiens* has his or her own unique chemistry. Despite this diversity, we all share certain important structural and biological features. For example, we are constructed from a host of different kinds of cells (blood, bone, nerve, muscle, etc.), most of which possess a nucleus containing our hereditary material—the chromosomes and their constituent genes, both of which are made from molecules of DNA (deoxyribonucleic acid) (see Fig. 1.1). Like our primeval ancestors we are mostly made of water—45–75 per cent depending upon age, build, and sex. In addition

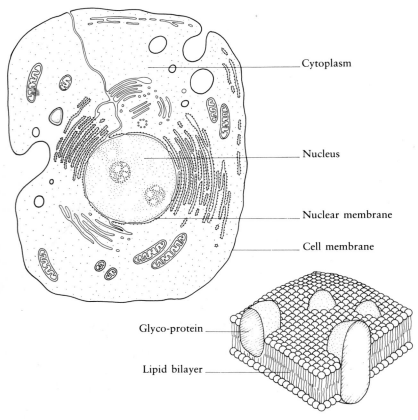

Fig. 1.1 A typical cell.

our cells contain substantial amounts of the non-metallic elements carbon, hydrogen, oxygen, nitrogen, sulphur, phosphorus, and chlorine; considerable quantities of the metallic elements sodium, potassium, and calcium; and small or trace amounts of 20 or so other chemical elements. These are mostly bound up in the molecules of carbohydrates (sugars), lipids (fats), proteins, and nucleic acids (DNA and RNA), which are the primary components of the cells, and most of the dynamic processes that occur within our cells involve these molecules. Molecules are composed of atoms that are held together by chemical bonds. A water molecule, for example, has two atoms of hydrogen and one atom of oxygen, and thus has the composition H_2O; its structure is depicted in Fig. 1.2. A molecule of glucose comprises six carbon atoms, twelve hydrogen atoms, and six

Water

Glucose

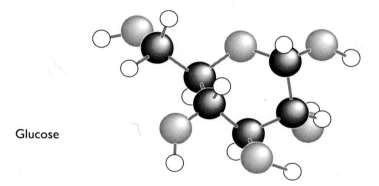

Fig. 1.2 Comparison of a molecule of water and a molecule of glucose.

oxygen atoms held together in a specific three-dimensional arrangement, also shown in Fig. 1.2. However, this same molecule of glucose is very small, with a diameter of only one-millionth of a millimetre. In contrast, a red blood cell is ten thousand times larger, with a diameter of around one hundredth of a millimetre. A human ovum is ten times larger still and is just about visible to the naked eye. Both types of cell contain millions of molecules. Biochemical processes are mainly under the control of a host of biological catalysts called enzymes (which are also proteins); these facilitate interconversions of chemical compounds, so that the processes occur up to a billion times faster than the corresponding chemical conversions would in a test tube. This intracellular biochemistry is separated from the extracellular environment by the cell membrane, and this comprises mainly a lipid bilayer of around 7.5–10 nanometres (i.e. billionths of a metre) thickness. The membrane provides structure but is also semipermeable, and thus allows nutrients and waste products respectively to pass into and out of the cell. Some molecules, including a number of glycoproteins (proteins with associated carbohydrate moieties) and certain enzymes, span the cell membrane and have important roles in intercellular communication and outside-to-inside communication.

The biological system of which our cells are a constituent part is in constant interaction with the environment: the air that we breathe, the fluids that we drink, the food that we eat, and the drugs that we take. Any of these external influences may change the exquisitely controlled biochemical processes that keep us alive and functioning normally.

Pharmacology is the science that seeks to identify the interactions of drugs with the various cell types, and to understand the resultant biochemical and physiological changes that occur. In a broader sense it is more valuable to consider changes produced by interactions of cells with any foreign substance—so-called xenobiotics (from the Greek *xenos*, strange, and *bios*, life). These include pollutants in the air and water, food additives and contaminants, as well as the drugs we take. We absorb these via our lungs, skin, or gastrointestinal tract; they are broken down (metabolized) mainly in the liver, and excreted via our skin, lungs, kidneys, and bowels. During these processes, biochemical and physiological changes occur, and these are usually a result of alterations in intercellular communication. So, in order to understand the effects of xenobiotics, we should first consider the normal modes of communication between cells.

Intercellular communication can occur in three main ways:

(a) neurotransmission, whereby a nerve cell passes a chemical signal on to another nerve cell or to a muscle cell;

(b) hormonal, whereby circulating hormones ('chemical messengers') are released from glands and carried by the blood stream to a distant organ; and

(c) autacoid, whereby local hormones are released and act on nearby cells.

Neurotransmission

A typical nerve cell (or neuron) is illustrated in Fig. 1.3. It comprises a cell body of varying diameter (5–100 micrometres, i.e. millionths of a metre)

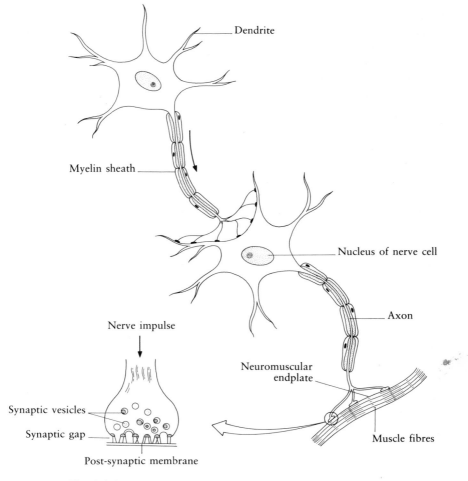

Fig. 1.3 Nerve axon, synapse, and neuromuscular endplate.

and a fibre or axon, which usually branches extensively into dendrites. In man the axon varies in length from less than a millimetre to almost a metre (e.g. in the spinal chord), and in diameter from 1–25 micrometres, although some of this thickness can include a non-continuous protein coat. This coat is termed the myelin sheath and functions as an electrical insulator.

At rest the neuron has different concentrations of ions (atoms or groups of atoms that carry an electrical charge because they have lost or gained electrons) on the inside to those in the surrounding fluid. Typical relative concentration values for several ions are shown in Fig. 1.4. There is a thin membrane (made up primarily of lipid) around the axon, and this is selectively permeable to potassium (K^+) and chloride (Cl^-) ions, and at

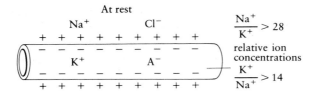

AT REST the axonal membrane is permeable to potassium ions (K^+) and chloride ions (Cl^-), but much less permeable to sodium ions (Na^+), and virtually impermeable to large (organic) anions (A^-). The relative ion concentrations outside and inside the axon are shown.

During the passage of a nerve impulse

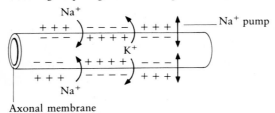

Axonal membrane

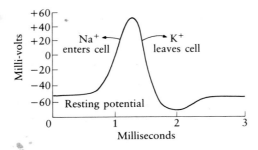

Fig. 1.4 Axonal ion conductance.

least 50–100 times less permeable to sodium (Na^+) than to potassium ions. There is a small excess of negative ions on the inside of the neuron, and of positive ions on the outside, and at rest there is an electrical potential difference of up to -85 millivolts. These properties are also possessed by most other cells—the difference between a nerve cell and these other cells is that the former are excitable.

Excitation of a neuron is caused by local changes in the concentrations of various neurotransmitter substances and/or certain ions, and as a result there occurs a selective in-rush of sodium ions via special sodium channels. This leads to a depolarization, in other words a rise in potential difference to around $+30$ millivolts, all within the space of a millisecond (a thousandth of a second). At this point the sodium channels close, and separate potassium channels open to allow an outflow of potassium ions and restoration of the original potential difference. The nerve impulse is thus propagated as a series of depolarizations and repolarizations. In order to attain its original state, the neuron must now pump out the excess sodium ions and allow the uptake of potassium ions, and this must be accomplished before it can accept another impulse.

There is no direct connection between nerve fibres or between nerve fibres and muscles or glands, and at the junction between these cells the electrical signal is converted into a chemical one. The electrical signal causes the release of a neurotransmitter substance, which moves across the gap between the two cells. For interneuronal communications this junction is known as a synapse, and for other cell types it is termed a neuroeffector junction.

The neurotransmitter binds to a specific receptor site, rather as a key fits into a lock, as depicted in Fig. 1.5. These receptors are usually glycoproteins of specific three-dimensional structure located on the surface of the post-synaptic cell membrane. Many drugs and other xenobiotics also fit into the various types of receptors: those that elicit a response are termed 'agonists', and those that block the receptor site without initiating a response are called 'antagonists'.

The neurotransmitter thus attaches itself to a receptor on the next neuron and initiates a new electrical impulse, or binds to a muscle end-plate or innervated gland and causes stimulation or inhibition. How these changes are effected is not completely understood, but alterations in cell membrane permeability to calcium, sodium, potassium, or chloride ions are probably involved. The neurotransmitter is then destroyed by the action of destructive enzymes or may be reabsorbed into the neural cell from which it was released.

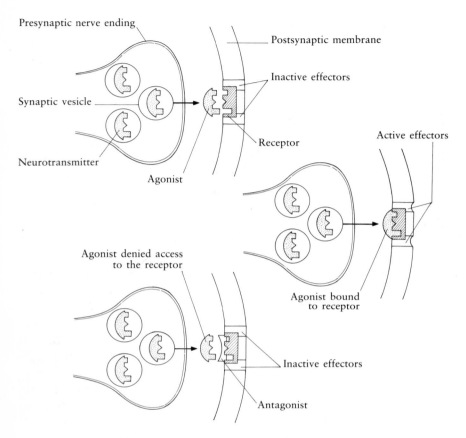

Fig. 1.5 Receptors: agonists and antagonists.

Many kinds of drug and other xenobiotics exert their effects by preventing or increasing the release of neurotransmitters, by binding to their receptors thus denying them access, by changing the permeability of the various cell membranes involved, by mimicking the action of the neurotransmitter, or by altering its re-uptake by the neuron. In order to understand these effects, we need to consider the normal functions of the main neurotransmitters.

Acetylcholine
This chemical is undoubtedly the most important neurotransmitter. It interacts with two sub-types of postsynaptic receptors—the so-called muscarinic and nicotinic receptors. The names reflect the fact that the

natural plant substances muscarine (from the fly agaric mushroom *Amanita muscaria*) and nicotine (from the tobacco plant *Nicotiana tabacum*) will compete with acetylcholine for binding at their respective receptors and also cause stimulation. A comparison of the structures of these substances is shown in Fig. 1.6.

Noradrenalin and adrenalin (the catecholamines)

At certain neuronal junctions, notably in the gut, lungs, and heart, excitation elicits the release of noradrenalin (a structural relative of the more familiar adrenalin); whilst stimulation of the adrenal glands (which lie just above the liver) produces adrenalin. These two neurotransmitters bind to so-called adrenoceptors (receptors for the catecholamines), of which at least three main types have been identified, and elicit a plethora of responses. These responses and those due to acetylcholine can best be explained pictorially as shown in Fig. 1.7.

Nerves leaving the brain and innervating all organs, but not skeletal muscles (which are under voluntary control), are part of the *autonomic nervous system*. Two types of nerves are identified, primarily on the basis of their anatomical origins (though there are also pharmacological differences): sympathetic and parasympathetic nerves. Our response to a threatening situation (the so-called 'fright–flight' reaction) provides a good example of the results of stimulation of the sympathetic nervous system. Adrenalin and noradrenalin are released and act upon the heart, lungs, gut, and peripheral blood vessels. As a result the heart rate increases, the bronchioles (numerous fine air passages in the lungs) are dilated (opened up) to allow for more efficient uptake of oxygen, and blood is diverted from the gut to the skeletal muscles. In addition, our pupils dilate, our hair may stand on end, and constriction of the peripheral blood vessels may lead to pallor.

In contrast, when we are relaxed, stimulation of the parasympathetic system by acetylcholine is predominant, and the heart rate falls while blood flow is diverted to the gut to facilitate, for example, digestion.

Clearly our normal functioning relies to a great extent upon a delicate balance of these two parts of the autonomic system. Any xenobiotic that can upset this balance will produce a pharmacological response, with resultant changes in overall biochemistry. Our awareness of what is happening within us depends upon the magnitude of these changes.

Hormones

The term hormone is usually reserved for chemical compounds released by

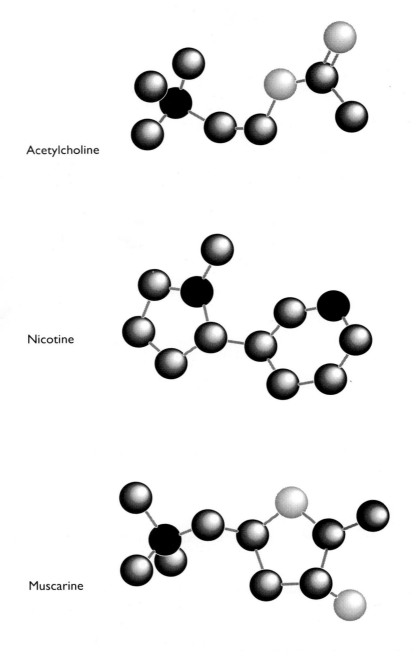

Fig. 1.6 Comparison of the structures of acetylcholine, nicotine, and muscarine.

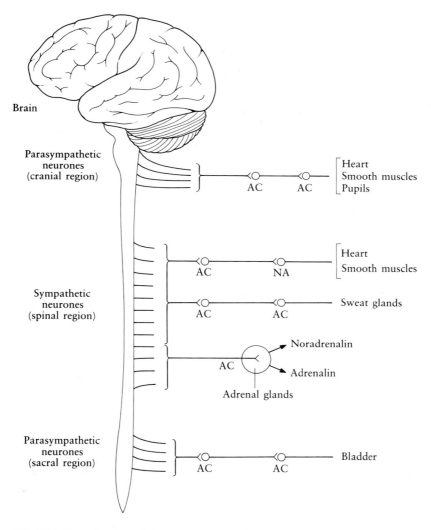

Brain

Parasympathetic
neurones
(cranial region)

AC   AC

Heart
Smooth muscles
Pupils

AC   NA

Heart
Smooth muscles

Sympathetic
neurones
(spinal region)

AC   AC

Sweat glands

AC

Noradrenalin

Adrenalin

Adrenal glands

Parasympathetic
neurones
(sacral region)

AC   AC

Bladder

Fig. 1.7 Organization of the nerves. AC and NA denote neuronal junctions
at which acetylcholine or noradrenalin are employed.

glands called endocrine glands, and carried in the bloodstream to distant
cells where they exert their effects. The hormone oxytocin is a good
example of this type, since it is released from the pituitary (a small gland at
the base of the brain), yet acts on the uterus and mammary glands. At the
full term of pregnancy it causes contraction of the uterus, which precedes
childbirth; it also induces lactation at the same time.

A second example is testosterone, which is produced by the testes, yet controls the development of the male sex organs, male secondary sexual characteristics (such as beard growth, deepening of the voice, etc.), and behaviour. Oxytocin is a peptide hormone, that is, it is constructed from amino acids, the basic building blocks of proteins, while testosterone is a steroid, a type of lipid, as is cholesterol.

Of more direct relevance to this book are the local hormones (or autacoids). Histamine and serotonin will be discussed now, and others will be mentioned in the main part of the book.

Histamine

Histamine is released from cells in the gastric mucosa, the lining of the stomach, in response to eating, and acts as a powerful stimulant of gastric acid production. It is also released from mast cells (one type of white blood cell) in the lungs and elsewhere in response to an allergic event, such as contact with grass pollen or house dust. The tightening of the bronchioles (bronchoconstriction) which causes an asthmatic attack and the rhinitis (runny nose) and watery eyes that accompany hayfever are two familiar manifestations of its effects.

Serotonin

Serotonin (or 5-hydroxytryptamine) is also found primarily in the gastric mucosa, but is also produced by certain neurons in the central nervous system. Indeed there is good evidence that serotonin acts as a neurotransmitter in many regions of the brain, and appears to be intimately involved with the control of sleep states and with vomiting. A deficiency of serotonin in the brain has also been implicated in migraine and depression.

Signal transduction

All of these chemical messengers convey a primary signal to a cell. Once they have interacted with their respective receptors, the signal must be translated into an event of some kind. This is known as signal transduction, and in Fig. 1.8 the main kinds of translation processes are depicted.

Many of the neurotransmitters have receptors that control a kind of 'gate' across a channel through the cell membrane. Normally the channel is closed, but, after binding of the neurotransmitter, there is a structural change and the 'gate' opens to allow small ions like sodium and chloride to pass through the channel and into the cell. Most of the non-steroidal

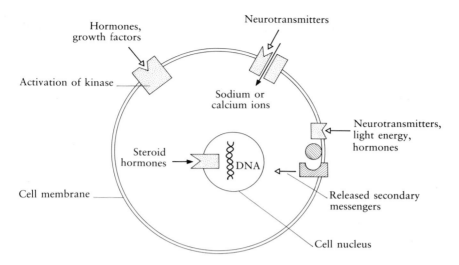

Fig. 1.8 Signal transduction.

hormones and growth factors (like insulin and oxytocin) have receptors that can activate enzymes known as tyrosine kinases. These control the level of activity of certain other key enzymes. A third type of receptor involves neither channels nor tyrosine kinases, but have associated with them so-called G-proteins which when activated can release a variety of 'secondary messengers' that convey a signal into the cell. Adrenalin and light impinging on the retina in the eye function in this way.

These secondary messengers include the chemical compounds cyclic adenosine monophosphate (cyclic AMP) and inositol triphosphate, both of which elicit the release of calcium ions from intracellular stores. The increased calcium ion levels then cause activation (or inhibition) of certain key enzymes.

Finally, the steroid hormones (like testosterone and the female hormones known as oestrogens) have no receptors on the outside of the cell, but pass through the cell membrane and bind to receptors inside the cell. Once bound, this receptor–hormone complex is transported into the nucleus of the cell and interacts with the hereditary material (DNA), triggering a burst of growth or differentiation. DNA acts as a blueprint for the production of RNA, which then acts as a blueprint for the production of new proteins and enzymes within the cytoplasm of the cell.

Our understanding of the fine details of these interactions is still at a fundamental stage, but for the purposes of this book it is only necessary to appreciate that almost all xenobiotics exert their effects by in some way affecting a cell receptor with consequent changes in cellular biochemistry. It is the ultimate pharmacological and physiological responses that have always been of particular interest to people, and why they have learnt to use plant and animal extracts for murder, magic, and medicine.

Murder

†

Toxic plant and animal products have been used for thousands of years in hunting, execution, and warfare. Usually, the poisonous extracts were smeared on arrows or spears, and the earliest reliable written evidence for such use appears in the Rig Veda, an ancient poetic work from the Vedic period in India (*c.* 1200 BC). The ancient Greek word *toxikon* originally meant 'poison for arrows'. Both Homer and Virgil mention the use of arrow poisons derived from natural sources. For example, in the *Odyssey*, Athena reports that when she first met Odysseus he 'was seeking the deadly poison [probably aconite] wherewith to anoint his bronze-tipped arrows'. Aconite was also the most widely used arrow poison in medieval Europe, and was still in use on the Iberian peninsula as late as the seventeenth century. Despite the potential of these toxins as agents of warfare and other murderous activities, they were originally intended as important hunting accessories. The arrow poisons of South America and Africa provide excellent examples of this.

Arrow poisons

In the sixteenth century explorers reported that the Indians of Brazil, Peru, Ecuador, and Colombia were using arrows tipped with *curari* or *woorali*—local names for what we now call 'curare'. This is a crude, dried extract of the plant *Chondrodendron tomentosum*, usually in admixture with various *Strychnos* species.

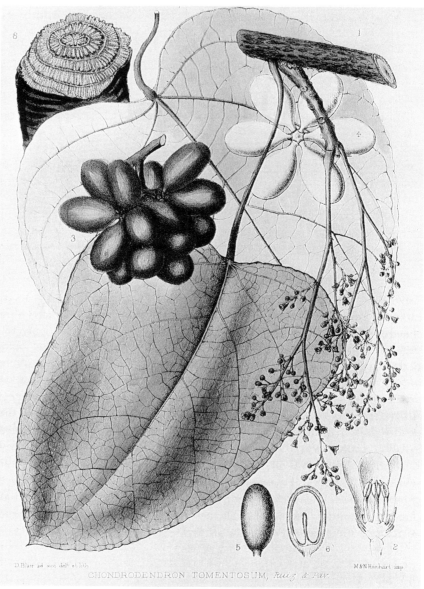

CHONDRODENDRON TOMENTOSUM, *Ruiz & Pav.*

Chrondrodendron tomentosum

Vivid accounts of the efficacy of these arrow poisons were related by, among others, the Spanish explorer Francisco de Orellano: 'the Indians killed another companion of ours ... and in truth, the arrow did not penetrate half a finger, but, as it had poison on it, he gave up his soul to our Lord'; and Sir Walter Raleigh: 'the party shot indureth the most insufferable torment ... and abideth a most ugly and lamentable death'.

But, in the main, fantastic and largely misleading tales reached Europe. In particular, myths arose about the modes of preparation of these poisons, and their efficacy was believed to be somehow related to the type of storage vessels used, i.e. 'tube', 'pot', or 'gourd' curares. In 1800 the explorers Humboldt and Bonpland gave the first accurate account of curare preparation: it involved making an aqueous extract of the bark from the vines with subsequent concentration to yield a tar-like mass. This was classified as 'one-tree' curare if a wounded monkey could make only one leap before expiring; 'three-tree' curare could be used to capture animals alive.

There was still total ignorance concerning the mode of action of the toxin until Charles Waterton began his experiments with animals in the 1820s. His crucial experiment involved a she-ass which appeared to expire ten minutes after he administered curare, but was then revived by artificial ventilation of its lungs using a bellows. The animal went on to make a full recovery, and the obvious implication was that curare caused death by asphyxiation. In 1844 the French physiologist Claude Bernard, using nerve–muscle preparations from frogs, confirmed that curare blocked transmission of nerve impulses to the muscles. Injection of the arrow poison into the blood stream thus caused death by respiratory failure (asphyxiation), because the chest and abdominal muscles were paralysed.

Much of the credit for the subsequent popularization and eventual clinical exploitation of curare must go to the American Richard Gill who spent much of the 1920s living with the Indians in Ecuador and learning how to prepare and use the toxin. On his return to the USA in 1938 he carried with him around 30 pounds of curare, but his attempts to excite the interest of the various drug companies met with total failure, and in desperation he set up his own curare business in California. An account of his adventures, *White Water and Black Magic*, was widely read, and eventually two drug companies, Squibb and Burroughs Wellcome, began experiments with curare.

Early attempts to use curare as a muscle relaxant were carried out in conjunction with ether as anaesthetic, and the experimental animals died of respiratory failure. In 1942 the Americans Griffiths and Johnson first

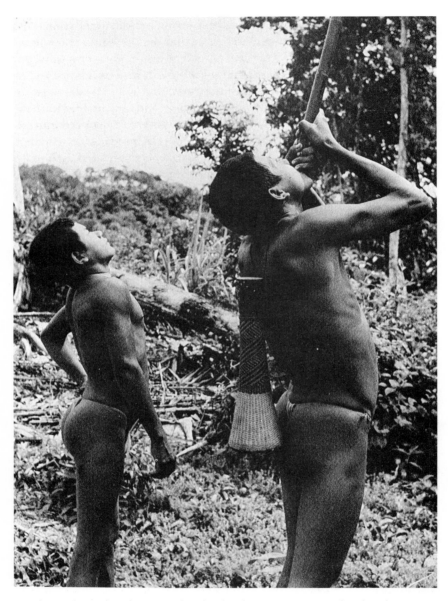

The Maku Indian hunters of Colombia have a reputation for their potent curare preparations. (From the personal collection of Professor Richard Evans Schultes, Emeritus Director, Botanical Museum of Harvard University.)

realized that artificial ventilation was necessary if the drug was to be used safely in conjunction with an anaesthetic. In the same year they went on to carry out dozens of successful operations on humans using the new strategy.

The most potent constituent of curare, tubocurarine, was isolated by Dr Harold King in 1935, but owing to lack of fresh material he was forced to use an old, dried specimen from the British Museum as his source. This sample had been stored in a tube, and that was why the major constituent of curare was christened 'tubocurarine'. The availability of reasonable quantities of tubocurarine from the work at Squibb and Burroughs Well-come allowed clinical evaluation to begin, and, as was usual at the time, the human guinea-pigs were company employees. Thus, Dr Frederick Prescott, Wellcome's director of clinical research, was one of the first to have himself injected with the new drug. The sensational press reports, for example, 'Doctor Died for Seven Minutes', helped to ensure a speedy entry of the drug into clinical use.

Supplies of curare still come from the South American jungles, though isolation and purification of tubocurarine takes place in the USA and Britain. The Indians continue to use the crude plant product as a highly effective arrow poison, even though firearms are now widely available. Interestingly, and fortunately for these native hunters, curare is poorly absorbed via the gastrointestinal tract, so consumption of the prey killed with the toxin is not hazardous.

Tubocurarine binds to the motor end-plate receptors and thus denies access to the neurotransmitter acetylcholine, with resultant paralysis of the muscles. For surgery it allows a reduction to be made in the amount of general anaesthetic required to achieve complete muscle relaxation, though the resultant paralysis of the respiratory muscles means that arti-ficial ventilation of the patient is necessary. Typically a dose of 20–30 mg produces a paralysis lasting for around 30 minutes.

A number of other toxins have been isolated from the various curare preparations used by South American Indians, and C-toxiferine, from *Strychnos toxifera*, is probably the most important after tubocurarine. It is about twenty-five times more potent than tubocurarine and has a longer duration of action when used in surgical practice, though both drugs have been largely superseded by other wholly synthetic neuromuscular blocking agents, such as pancuronium and atracurium. Like tubocurarine these have a rigid molecular structure with two positively charged nitrogen atoms held in a similar spatial arrangement to that found in tubocurarine (see Fig. 2.1). This allows them to bind to the same acetylcholine receptor and thus mimic the biological activity of tubocurarine, because the dis-

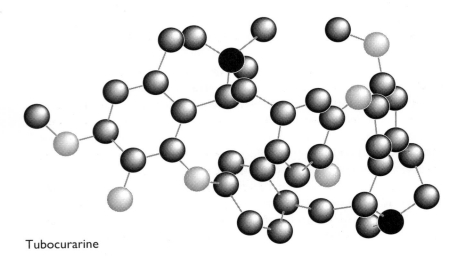

Tubocurarine

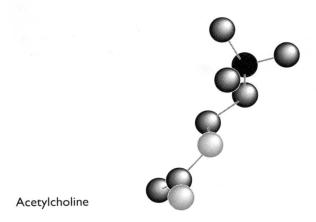

Acetylcholine

Fig. 2.1 Comparison of the structures of acetylcholine and tubocurarine.

tance between the two cationic centres (N^+ to N^+ distance) is approximately the same. The major advantage of the newer synthetic agents is their shorter duration of activity, and the induced paralysis is thus more easily regulated.

In Africa the arrow poisons were usually based upon extracts of various *Strophanthus* species, and the great Victorian explorer David Livingstone was among the first to describe the native use of these plants. The major active principle from *Strophanthus hispidus*, strophanthidin, has an effect on the heart similar to that elicited by digitalis from the foxglove (discussed in Chapter 3). A toxic dose produces nausea and vomiting, and a marked lowering of the heart rate and various heartbeat arrhythmias.

David Livingstone also noted that a related plant species, *Strophanthus gratus*, yielded an arrow poison that could stop even an elephant in its tracks. The active ingredient, ouabain, has similar effects to strophanthidin, but at a much lower dose. Just as with curare (and in contrast to digitalis) both arrow poisons are poorly absorbed via the gastrointestinal tract, so prey killed in this way is generally safe to eat.

The mode of action of these cardiac glycosides is different from that of curare. They all inhibit the functioning of a sodium/potassium ion pump that is needed for maintenance of the normal ion balance in heart muscle cells. One consequence of this is that the concentration of sodium ions inside the cell increases, and this triggers a mobilization of calcium ions which can, at therapeutic doses, result in more efficient muscular contraction. This effect is of considerable value in the treatment of congestive heart failure and of heart arrhythmias. In both states the circulation of blood is impaired, and, if not treated, the tissues (especially the brain) become starved of oxygen. Administration of cardiac glycosides increases the force and efficiency of contraction of heart muscle, and at the same time the heart rate is slowed. Cardiac output is thus made more efficient, and this is vital if the heart failure is to be reversed.

In larger, toxic, doses the cardiac glycosides cause serious disruptions in the ionic balance of the heart muscle cells, producing arrhythmias and ultimately cardiac arrest. The therapeutic benefits of cardiac glycosides from the foxglove were first described by William Withering in the eighteenth century, and his studies will be described in Chapter 3.

Classical poisons I: the tropane alkaloids

In addition to their use as arrow poisons, toxic plant products were also much used for executions. One of the best documented examples of a mass execution involved the use of the tree *Antiaris toxicaria* (the upas tree), a native of tropical Asia. The sap of this tree contains cardiac glycosides, though legend maintained that a toxic vapour emanated from the tree, and this is graphically represented in the painting by Francis Danby, entitled *The Upas Tree*. In 1776 one of the local 'kings' of Java expressed his displeasure with thirteen unfaithful concubines by having them executed with sap from the upas tree. They were tied to posts with their breasts bared, and the executioner administered the poison using an awl-like instrument to make an incision. They all died within minutes in the utmost agony. The same plant extract was also used to poison the wells of the Dutch colonists, and although subsequent pharmacological investigation suggested a use for the major constituent, antiarin, as a heart drug to rival digitalis, its great toxicity has precluded its clinical use.

The crudeness of this method of execution would have shocked the expert poisoners of the ancient world, who were masters (or, more often than not, mistresses) of the toxic arts. They could select a poison that would take days or even months to take effect, thus ensuring that the unfaithful or ineffectual spouse or lover would not suspect the reason for his or her lingering illness. On occasions when a more rapid result was required, a stronger dose or more powerful poison could be prescribed. When Cleopatra decided to take her life she first of all experimented with various plant extracts, using her slaves for acute toxicity tests. Extracts from henbane (*Hyoscyamus niger*) and deadly nightshade (*Atropa belladonna*) produced a rapid but painful effect; strychnine was also quick, but left the face contorted in death (the so-called *risus sardonicus*). However, the asp's venom allowed a rapid and tranquil passage into the afterworld.

The two plants just mentioned are members of the Solanaceae family (as are the potato, the tomato, and tobacco), and were an essential source of poisons, hallucinogens, and medicines for the ancient pharmacists. A single berry from deadly nightshade incorporated into food or drink contained enough toxins to cause death; and the long list of victims who suffered at the hands of Livia (wife of the Emperor Augustus) and Agrippina (wife of Claudius) is a testament to the efficacy of belladonna. Augustus apparently knew of his wife's evil intentions and thwarted her attempts on his life by preparing all of his own food and drink. However, she finally succeeded by injecting poison into the figs growing on his personal tree.

Juice from belladonna berries when squeezed into the eyes produces dilation of the pupils, and was thus much used by Renaissance ladies to impart a 'doe-eyed beauty' look—hence the name 'belladonna' (Italian for 'beautiful woman'). The main constituent of the berries, atropine, was

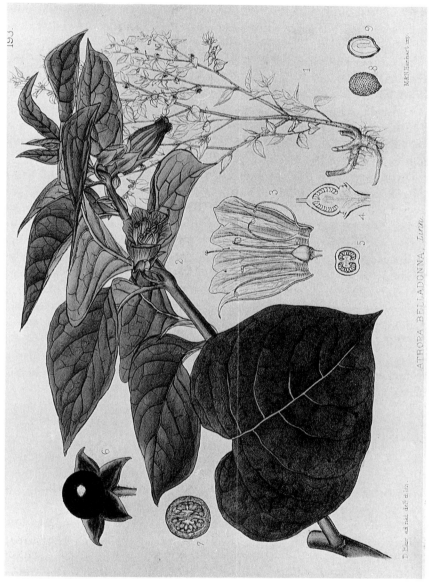

Atropa belladonna.

until quite recently used for the same purpose in ophthalmology, since a fully dilated pupil allows a ready examination of the retina. It has now been superseded by safer synthetic analogues, though it is still widely used to dry up bronchial and other secretions before surgery.

The other plant mentioned above, henbane, was also much used by the criminal classes, and Pliny noted that as little as four leaves taken in a drink would put the recipient 'beside himself'. The prime constituent here is hyoscine (scopolamine). and in controlled doses this has a useful sedative and soothing effect familiar to anyone who has received it as a premedication before surgery. Its involvement in witchcraft and sorcery will be described in Chapter 2.

A third member of the Solanaceae family, the mandrake (*Mandragora officinarum*), also contains hyoscine, and it has the most fantastic folklore associated with its use. It is indigenous to countries bordering the Mediterranean Sea, and in appearance its Y-shaped root can resemble the human form. According to the 'doctrine of signatures' first proposed by the alchemist Paracelsus, the magical or curative properties of a plant could be predicted from its appearance. Hence, a plant that resembled the human form would favour reproduction of that form. So the mandrake has always been associated with enhancement of fertility. An early example of this belief can be seen in Genesis 30:14, where the childless Rachel implores her extremely fecund sister Leah to 'Give me, I pray thee, of thy son's mandrakes' after Reuben had found some in a field of wheat. In the following lines by John Donne, we can also see further evidence of this belief, and also its associations with the black arts:

> *Go, and catch a falling star,*
> *Get with child a mandrake root,*
> *Tell me, where all the past years are,*
> *Or who cleft the devil's foot.*

The root also possessed supposed aphrodisiac properties, and the plant was associated with Aphrodite, the Greek goddess of love.

The major problem facing those who wished to use the mandrake was collection of the root. In the third century BC the Greek pharmacist Theophrastus described special precautions for collection which involved tracing a circle three times around the plant with a sword and then cutting it while facing west. Later, Pliny the Elder also advised keeping to windward to avoid the foul stench of the uprooted plant.

As the root became more highly prized, especially in medieval Europe, so the herbalists invented ever more fanciful (and deterrent) legends.

Collection of a mandrake root depicted in a sixteenth century manuscript illustration. (Wellcome Institute Library, London.)

Typical of these was the one that warned of the terrible shriek that issued from the mandrake as it was pulled from the ground. This sound was so awful that the collector upon hearing it would die. To avoid this fate, a dog was to be used (with a rope around its neck and attached to the plant) to uproot the mandrake, while the collector blocked his ears with wax.

These legends were widely believed, and the precautions were thought to be essential if the demons associated with the root were to be avoided. The use of a dog can be traced as far back as the first century AD, when the Jewish historian Josephus described this mode of collection in conjunction with a liberal sprinkling of the plant with female urine and menstrual blood. References to the legends are also common in Shakespeare's plays. In *Romeo and Juliet*, Juliet feared the 'shrieks like mandrakes, torn out of the earth,/That living mortals, hearing them, run mad' (IV, iii); in *Henry VI (part II)*, the Duke of Suffolk yearns to revenge the murder of the Duke of Gloucester: 'Would curses kill, as doth the mandrake's groan' (III, ii); and finally in *Macbeth*: 'Or have we eaten on the insane root/That takes the reason prisoner?' (I, iii). But perhaps the best literary reference is found in an anonymous poem from the Middle Ages:

> *Then on the still night air,*
> *The bark of a dog is heard,*
> *A shriek! A groan!*
> *A human cry. A trumpet sound,*
> *The mandrake root lies captive on the ground.*

However, the shriek was not all that would kill, for fermented mandrake root was a favourite of the Renaissance poisoners, like Cesare Borgia. If one detected the symptoms of poisoning (trembling, stomach pains, yellowing of the eyes, etc.), there was an antidote, but the long list of essential ingredients (honey, butter, oatmeal, mint leaves, anise, nutmeg, fennel seed, clove bark, ginger, cinnamon, celery, radish, dill, etc.) provided something of a challenge for those wishing to avoid the almost inevitable sequelae—epileptic seizures and death. Dr Crippen also employed hyoscine as a poison, and he was able to buy the poison from a pharmacy in New Oxford Street.

Yet another of the Solanaceae family, *Datura stramonium* (and many other *Datura* species), was also intimately involved with crime and seduction. It is almost ubiquitous, and the seeds and the berries are particularly poisonous, with hyoscine again a major constituent. In toxic doses it ensured insensibility before an almost painless death, but if the extract was given in smaller amounts it had a sedative (and possibly aphrodisiac) effect. In this way the white slavers were able to abduct young virgins, though, in apposition to this, Hindu whores in the sixteenth century wreaked a kind of revenge on their clients by drugging them with *Datura* extracts, thus minimizing the demands on their services. Thieves in Colombia have recently resorted to using extracts of *Datura* species as the basis of an intoxicating mixture that is sprayed into the face of a victim. The mixture apparently produces a state of submission and a complete loss of memory, thus facilitating the theft and preventing subsequent recognition.

The toxic effects of *Datura* were probably responsible for the losses suffered by Mark Antony's army in AD 36. During his campaign against the Pathans in Asia Minor, his troops were forced to eat unfamiliar plants, and they 'ate of one plant that killed them after driving them mad'. A more deliberate use of this species for poisoning was prevalent in ancient Colombia, where nursing mothers practised infanticide by smearing their nipples with *Datura* extracts. The Chibcha tribe (also Colombian) administered poison from *Datura aurea* to wives and slaves of recently deceased potentates before burying them alive. The Spanish explorer Quesada reported in 1537 that forty of his party began raving while in a Chibcha village. Fortunately he discovered the reason—food poisoned with *Datura* extracts—and his men subsequently recovered.

In more recent times, *Datura stramonium* achieved a notoriety in the New World when some of the early settlers near Jamestown, Virginia, mistook it for spinach and narrowly avoided death. The plant subsequently became known as Jamestown weed, or jimsonweed, and was used for a wide variety of medicinal purposes, including the treatment of mania, epilepsy, and melancholy. In the nineteenth century it was even sold in the form of herbal cigarettes by the Spanish Cigarette Company, and these were said to bring relief to those suffering from bronchial asthma and other respiratory conditions. A modern equivalent of this is the drug ipratropium (Atrovent), which is a synthetic structural analogue of atropine, and is an effective anti-asthmatic drug when given by inhalation.

Atropine was first isolated in 1831 and a water-soluble salt (atropine methonitrate) was introduced into ophthalmology in 1902. Hyoscine was first used clinically in 1910 as a premedication (Omnopon). Both these drugs exert their actions through a selective blockade on the muscarinic class of acetylcholine receptors, and their pharmacology and long association with witchcraft and magic will be described in Chapter 2.

Trials by ordeal

In primitive societies, when a person was accused of a crime they were

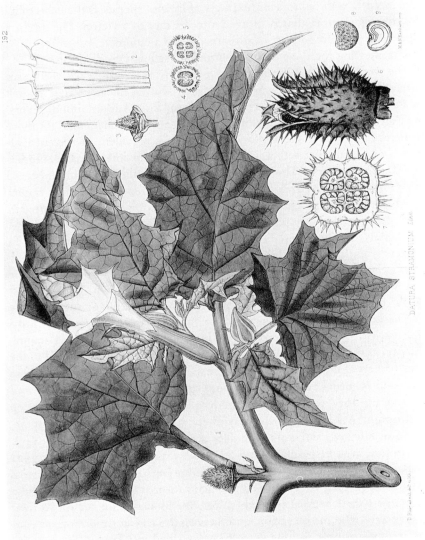

Datura stramonium.

often subjected to a trial by ordeal involving the administration of a toxic plant extract. The subsequent death of the victim implied guilt, while survival implied innocence. The trick was to consume the brew rapidly, for the powerful emetic properties of the toxins would then ensure rapid expulsion in the vomit. A truly innocent person might well do this, while a guilty person would probably sip the brew, thus allowing absorption of the poison via the gastrointestinal tract. However, this supposition ignores interference by the trial judges, who probably predetermined the outcome of the trial by selecting the appropriate dose to ensure survival or death.

Two plants which have a long association with this kind of ordeal ceremony are *Tanghinia venenifera* and *Physostigma venenosa*. Seeds of the former contain cardiac glycosides and were widely used in Madagascar until the French took over in 1883. They were appalled by the barbarity of the trials, and ordered the destruction of all *Tanghinia* trees.

Physostigma venenosa occurs in parts of West Africa, especially near the Calabar Coast, and its fruit is usually known as the Calabar bean. This contains a substance called physostigmine (or eserine), which has an important place in clinical medicine. Its discovery was, like many other such discoveries, intimately involved with the missionary service. In around 1840 a British missionary called William Daniell first observed that the Efik people were using extracts of the Calabar bean, known locally as esere, in trials by ordeal. His report was read to the Ethnological Society of Edinburgh in 1846, and stated:

> *The condemned person, after swallowing a certain portion of the liquid, is ordered to walk about until its effects become palpable. If, however, after the lapse of a definite period, the accused should be so fortunate as to throw the poison from off his stomach, he is considered innocent, and allowed to depart unmolested.*

The poison was also used in a more straightforward way in executions, and the kings of Old Calabar were usually buried in the company of hundreds of men, women, and children, who were decapitated, given esere, or simply buried alive. Even in recent times, the extracts have been used for the divination of witches. Thus, the anthropologist Donald Simmons wrote in 1956 of his encounters with the Efik people:

> *The Efik believe that the esere possesses the power to reveal witchcraft. A suspected person is given eight of the beans ground and added to water as a drink. If he is guilty, his mouth shakes and mucus comes from his nose. His innocence is proved if he lifts his*

right hand and then regurgitates. If the poison continues to affect the suspect after he has established his innocnce, he is given a concoction of excrement mixed in water which has been used to wash the external genitalia of a female.

The similarity of this account to that given by Daniell is obvious.

The second phase in the exploitation of esere took place at the Edinburgh Medical School. This famous institution had its origins in a plan by local physicians to create a herb garden that would supply their drug needs, and a long association between botany and medicine thus began. The first professor of botany was appointed in 1676, and the majority of the physicians were also accomplished botanists. One of these, John Hutton Balfour, was the first to provide a description of *Physostigma venenosa*, in 1846, and the plant was at that time growing (from seed supplied by the missionaries) in the Royal Botanic Garden in Edinburgh.

Toxicological studies began in the 1850s and were reported in the *Monthly Journal of Medicine* in 1855. The author of this report was Robert Christison, who was at that time professor of materia medica. Initially he experimented with animals and demonstrated that the ultimate cause of death was respiratory failure, though this was primarily due to paralysis of heart muscle rather than of the respiratory and abdominal muscles as occurs with curare. Not satisfied with his animal experiments, he did what all true pioneers of drug research do, and tried esere himself.

At first he only consumed one-eighth of a seed (*c*. 0.35 g) and suffered merely a slight numbness in the extremities, so he proceeded to take double that dose. A slight giddiness occurred after fifteen minutes, but he none the less continued with his morning ablutions. The giddiness became rapidly more marked, and becoming alarmed he 'took immediate means for getting quit of it [the poison], by swallowing the shaving water I had just been using'. Within forty minutes he had to take to his bed with a feeble pulse and extreme pallor, but with his mental faculties unimpaired. Two hours after consuming the seed, he became drowsy and slept for two hours, waking to find that his heart was still beating feebly. After a further hour, and a cup of strong coffee, his heart was restored to its normal state, though he remained 'so giddy as to be glad to betake myself to the sofa for the evening'.

In passing, it is worth recording that this experience did not deter him from other toxicological studies, since at the age of 78 he experimented with cocaine, walking long distances and clambering up mountains, to demonstrate the fatigue- and hunger-relieving properties of the drug.

One of Christison's assistants, Thomas Fraser, extended his studies, showing that small doses of esere mainly affected the nerves of the spinal chord, and that death (if it occurred) was due to paralysis of the respiratory muscles. With larger doses the heart was involved, and death was ultimately due to heart failure. But his major contribution was the discovery that instillation of a seed extract into the eye produced 'a copious secretion of tears, and in about five minutes a distinct contraction of the pupil confined to the side of application'. This effect was clearly the opposite of that produced by atropine, and this led Fraser to a further study, in which he demonstrated that the lethal effect of the bean extract could be prevented by the administration of atropine.

Work on the ophthalmic properties of esere continued under the direction of Douglas Robertson, who was an ophthalmic surgeon at the Edinburgh Royal Infirmary. He confirmed that the extract would counteract the effects of atropine, and he suggested that it derived its actions via stimulation of the ciliary nerves, the nerves responsible for controlling the muscles of the eyeball. He recommended use of the extract for the treatment of photophobia and paralysis of the ciliary muscles, but failed to appreciate its potential use in the treatment of glaucoma. This is a disorder of the eye in which the intraocular pressure is too high, thus causing damage to the optic nerve and leading ultimately to blindness.

In 1864 the major constituent of the Calabar bean had been isolated in pure form by Jobst and Hesse, and they named it physostigmine. The actual structure of the compound was not completely elucidated until 1925, but samples of pure physostigmine were available for ophthalmic use in the 1870s. In 1875 Ludwig Laqueur used it for the treatment of glaucoma, having noted that it would reduce intraocular pressure. From these hesitant beginnings, and despite the advent of wholly synthetic drugs, physostigmine became one of the most important drugs for the treatment of glaucoma.

A further major development occurred in 1906, when Anderson demonstrated that physostigmine would still cause contraction of the pupil, even if the local nerves were cut, though this effect vanished if the severed nerves were allowed to degenerate. This suggested the release of a chemical transmitter substance from non-degenerate nerve-endings, and that this substance was modified in some way by physostigmine. The involvement of acetylcholine as a neurotransmitter was not finally established until 1926, primarily due to the efforts of the Englishman Henry Dale and the Austrian Otto Loewi. They shared the Nobel prize for their work in 1936. One of the main features of its mode of action was its short biological lifetime, and Otto Loewi showed that the destruction of acetylcholine was probably due to the presence of an enzyme. The potentiating effect of physostigmine was thus due to inhibition of this enzyme.

All of this has been substantiated more recently, and the enzyme, acetylcholinesterase, has been the subject of exhaustive structural and mechanistic investigations. An understanding of the mode of action of physostigmine has led to two very different applications. For the first of these we have to return to the work of Frederich Jolly on the disease myasthenia gravis. This is a chronic condition which is characterized by muscular weakness during exertion, and is often first apparent in the eyelid muscles. Jolly was professor of medicine at the University of Strasbourg and he spent the best part of twenty years studying myasthenia gravis and related conditions. He suspected a disturbance in the chemistry of the muscles or in the nerves that activated them, and in 1894 he suggested that physostigmine, and other drugs that have a tonic effect on muscles, might be used in treatment. But it was not until 1934 that Mary Walker first used the drug to treat patients, and thus produced what became known as the 'miracle of St Alpheges'. She believed that the effects of the disease were similar to those caused by curare poisoning, for which physostigmine was an antidote. Her first patient at the Woolwich hospital was a woman of 56 who was admitted with classic symptoms of myasthenia gravis: 'She was unable to hold her shopping bag, and her head used to fall forwards when she knelt to do the hearth.' After a course of twenty-six injections of physostigmine the patient was much improved. Other patients were similarly treated either with physostigmine or a synthetic derivative called neostigmine, though the latter was thought too expensive for general use, 'an ampoule containing 0.5 mg of the drug being ninepence'.

Although it is not known what actually causes myasthenia gravis, it has now been established that persons suffering from the condition produce antibodies to their own acetylcholine receptors. These bind to the receptors and destroy them (just as if they were foreign proteins), and although new receptors are produced they are present in insufficient numbers to allow an efficient interaction with acetylcholine to occur. Physostigmine and neostigmine extend the biological lifetime of the neurotransmitter by preventing its destruction, and thus increase the chances of its interaction with the residual receptors. Both drugs are still much used for the treatment of this debilitating, though mercifully rare disease. More recently physostigmine has been shown to significantly reduce the memory loss experienced by sufferers of Alzheimer's disease, but it is too soon to tell whether the drug will have genuine clinical value in the treatment of this disease.

Inhibition of the enzyme acetylcholine esterase was also shown to be a key feature in the mode of action of the organophosphorus insecticides, like malathion, and the so-called carbamate insecticides, like carbaryl. These insecticides have structural homologies with physostigmine, and certainly the insects suffer a similar fate to the one experienced by the recipients of esere. None of these agents causes irreversible inhibition of the human enzyme, and with time it recovers its biological activity. However, in the mid-1930s certain organophosphorus agents produced by the German company I. G. Farben were shown to cause rapid and irreversible inhibition of the enzyme acetylcholinesterase. Not surprisingly the potential use of these compounds as neurotoxic agents (nerve gases) was recognized, and around 2000 compounds were produced and screened for activity between 1938 and 1944. The most active agents, like tabun, were produced in vast tonnages during the war. However, the Germans believed that the Allies also possessed these chemical weapons, so they were never used, which is just as well since as little as 1 mg of tabun, absorbed through the skin can kill an adult within twenty minutes.

The study of esere has clearly been of great value as an aid to understanding neurotransmission, and several clinically and agriculturally useful agents have emerged; but man has also taken a primitive poison and used it to design a much more potent contemporary poison.

Other modern insecticides have arisen from folklore, and the familiar 'derris dust' actually has a long association with fish poisoning in primitive societies. Local fishermen in the Far East and South America macerate plants of the *Derris* species (Far East) or of the *Lonchocarpus* species (South America), then fling the extracts into the water, thus paralysing the fish, which float to the surface. An even simpler means of administration involves chewing the plants then spitting the soggy mass into the water. Alternatively, in Melanesia and Polynesia, fishermen deposit a wet mass of derris leaves in depressions on the reef and then wait for passing fish to become stunned.

The Australian equivalent of this practice involves dropping leaves of the shrub *Duboisia hopwoodii* into water holes. This is said to kill fish and even emus, though only plants gathered in certain locations in central Australia were effective. Aborigines living on the eastern edge of the great central desert chewed leaves of the local *Duboisia* species for their stimulant effects. Recent chemical analysis has shown that the former subspecies of *hopwoodii* contains a predominance of the relatively toxic alkaloid nornicotine, while the latter subspecies contain primarily the stimulant nicotine.

The Aborigines prepared their *Duboisia* quids (for chewing), known as pituri, from sun-dried leaves. These were pulverized or chewed to produce a finely divided state, and then this mass was mixed with alkaline ash. This released the nicotine from the vegetable matrix and facilitated absorption of the drug through cell membranes. This mode of preparation and consumption is very similar to that employed by South American indians when using coca leaves (rich in cocaine) (see Chapter 2). This is clearly of great ethnopharmacological interest. Two cultures that were far removed geographically devised almost identical methods for obtaining their stimulants.

Marine toxins

Although man has probably used toxic plants to poison fishes for thousands of years, certain fish species have been poisoning man since he first became a fisherman. The puffer fish and other members of the family Tetraodontoidea, such as the globe fish and the porcupine fish, contain the deadly neurotoxin tetrodotoxin. The ancient Egyptians certainly knew about the puffer fish, since it is depicted on the tomb of the Pharaoh Ti (*c.* 2500 BC), and accounts dating from the time of the Han dynasty in China (200 BC to AD 220) clearly acknowledged that the fugu (or puffer) fish was poisonous. A later Chinese treatise entitled *Studies on the Origin of Diseases*, by Chaun Yanfang, (*c.* AD 600) identified the liver, ovaries, and roe (eggs) as the most toxic parts of the fish, and deliberate consumption of these parts was not an uncommon method of suicide in medieval China and Japan.

One of the first 'modern' accounts of the effects of fugu poisoning was recorded by Captain James Cook in 1774. He was on his second circumnavigation of the globe, when on 8 September he was presented with a fish that had not hitherto been seen by his naturalist. The latter duly made his drawings and other examinations, then Cook had the fish prepared for dinner. Fortunately neither of them did more than taste the liver and roe of the specimen, but the aftermath was none the less dramatic. Cook gave the following account of their experiences:

About three to four o'clock in the morning we were seized with most extraordinary weakness in all our limbs attended with numbness of sensation like that caused by exposing one's hands and feet to the fire after having been pinched much by the frost. I had almost lost the sense of feeling nor could I distinguish between light and heavy objects, a quart pot full of water and a feather was the same in my hand. We each took a vomit and after that a sweat which gave great relief. In the morning one of the pigs which had eaten the entrails was found dead. In the morning when the natives came aboard and saw the fish hanging up they immediately gave us to understand it was by no means to be eaten, expressing the utmost abhorrence of it and yet no one was observed to do this when it was sold or even after it was bought.

Whether the natives were trying to murder the foreigners is open to conjecture, but they were clearly very lucky to survive, for the lethal dose for man is probably similar to that for the mouse, i.e. around 10 micrograms per kilogram of body weight by injection (a bit more for the oral route). A similar tale was told by the Mexican historian Francisco Xavier Clavijero. Four soldiers found some leftovers from a native meal made from the puffer fish *Sphoerroides lobatus* (botete), which also contains tetrodotoxin. One of the soldiers ate a small piece of the fish liver and another merely chewed a small portion without swallowing it. None the less they were both dead within an hour.

Such poisoning is not of historical interest only, since several people are poisoned each year in the USA through eating puffer fish, and in Japan the problem is much more serious, because fugu is a delicacy. Great care must be taken in the preparation and cooking of the fish, and the chef must hold a licence before a restaurant can include fugu on the menu. The attraction seems to lie in the delicate flavour that traces of tetrodotoxin impart to food or drink, and there is a great temptation to use small portions of the fish for this purpose. A most apposite commentary on this practice appeared in a recent issue of *Trends in Pharmacological Sciences*:

The pleasures of fugu are ambiguous, being both gustatory and tactile. The presence of traces of tetrodotoxin in the food apparently leads to a delicious tingling sensation in the extremities accompanied by a feeling of warmth and euphoria. The first sign that something is going very, very wrong is the appearance of the same sensation in areas not extreme and the disappearance of the euphoria.

As to the mode of poisoning, tetrodotoxin halts nerve transmission by deactivating the uptake of sodium ions via the sodium channels in neuronal membranes, thus upsetting the delicate balance of sodium and potassium ions needed for signal transmission. Death is usually due to respiratory failure, and an understanding of the pharmacology of the toxin has allowed its use as a research tool for the investigation of modes of neurotransmission, and as a model for the design of less complex modulating drugs. For example, the use of tetrodotoxin and other neurotoxins has led to a greater understanding of the structures of sodium channels and the various 'gating' mechanisms. The sodium channel is thought to exist in three conformational states: a non-electrically-conducting resting state, a conducting state, and a non-conducting inactivated state. A pictorial representation of the acetylcholine receptor and its sodium channel is shown in Fig. 2.2.

Another marine toxin with human associations is palytoxin from seaweeds of the *Palythoa* genus. These are especially prevalent in the Caribbean and around Hawaii, and natives of the Hawaiian islands used to smear extracts from these seaweeds on to their spears for hunting and warfare. Palytoxin was first isolated in 1968, and complete elucidation of its structure was carried out during the 1970s. It is presently the most complex known molecule that is not a carbohydrate or protein and also the most toxic one of marine origin: the lethal dose for a mouse is of the order of 50–100 nanograms per kilogram of body weight. It depolarizes all excitable tissues thus far studied, including heart muscle, nerve axons, skeletal muscle, and smooth muscle (as in the gut), and it also causes rupture of red blood cells by precipitating rapid egress of potassium ions. These effects are apparently due to the induction of pores in the excitable membranes and an enhancement of the permeabilities of various ions.

Marine snails of the genus *Conus* exhibit perhaps the most exotic array of strategies for poisoning their prey and their predators, but there is little evidence for their use by man. They produce a variety of so-called conotoxins (and other toxins), all of which are polypeptides, and together they lead to total muscle paralysis. α-Conotoxin blocks the acetylcholine receptor on the postsynaptic site, while ω-conotoxin blocks transmitter release

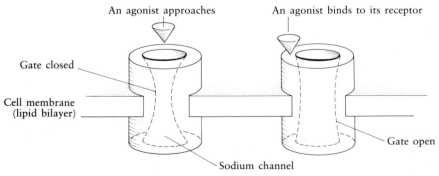

Fig. 2.2 The acetylcholine receptor and its sodium channel.

from the presynaptic site. Finally, μ-conotoxin selectively inhibits the functioning of the sodium channels of skeletal muscles, thus preventing excitation.

Any of these marine toxins would make ideal arrow poisons, and it is probably the relative inaccessibility of the creatures that has precluded their use for this purpose. These difficulties are less obvious with terrestrial creatures, and reptiles in particular have been widely used as sources of toxins.

Reptilian toxins

Most witches' brews, both fictional and real, contained fragments of reptiles—'eye of newt, and toe of frog'—and many reptiles can produce toxic secretions to deter predators. For example, the Californian newt *Taricha torosa* was known to produce a highly poisonous deterrent substance. In the 1960s pure toxin was isolated for the first time (12 mg from 100 kg of newt eggs), and structure elucidation provided the surprising result that this so-called tarichatoxin was in fact identical to tetrodotoxin. To give some idea of the potency of this relatively widespread toxin, a comparison with other well known poisons is instructive. The data shown are in the form of the minimum lethal dose per kilogram of body weight for the mouse:

Poison	Source	Lethal dose (micrograms)
Botulinus toxin	*Clostridium botulinus*	0.03
Tetanus toxin	*Clostridium tetani*	0.07
Cobra neurotoxin	*Naja naja*	0.3
Tetrodotoxin	Puffer fish	8–20
Curare or strychnine	*Strychnos* species	500
Samandarine	*Salamandra maculosa*	1500
Sodium cyanide		10 000

Among the most toxic amphibians are frogs of the genera *Phyllobates* and *Dendrobates*, which inhabit western Colombia and parts of Panama and Costa Rica. Their toxins have a long and interesting ethnopharmacological history. The frogs secrete their poison when under stress, such as when taken by a predator, and the natives use these toxins as arrow poisons.

One of the first accounts of this was given by Captain Charles Stuart Cochrane, a British naval officer who explored Colombia in 1823–4. He wrote:

Those who use poison catch the frogs in the woods, and confine them in a hollow cane, where they regularly feed them until they want the poison, when they take one of the unfortunate reptiles and pass a pointed piece of wood down his throat, and out at one of his legs. This torture makes the poor frog perspire very much, especially on the back, which becomes covered with white froth; this is the most powerful poison that he yields, and in this they dip or roll the points of their arrows, which will preserve their destructive power for a year. Afterwards, below this white substance, appears a yellow oil, which is carefully scraped off, and retains its deadly influence for four to six months, according to the goodness (as they say) of the frog. By this means, from one frog sufficient poison is obtained for about fifty arrows.

More recent anthropological surveys fully support this description, and in the 1960s structure elucidation of the toxins was carried out at the National Institute for Health in Washington DC, by Witcop, Daly, and their co-workers. At least 200 structures have now been identified, and most of these toxins interfere in some way or other with neurotransmission. One of the most potent is batrachotoxin, which is about five times more potent than tetrodotoxin and comes from the frog *Phyllobates aurotaenia*. Some 7000 frogs were collected in order to obtain enough toxin for the chemical and pharmacological studies. Batrachotoxin, in marked contrast to tetrodotoxin, enhances the transport of sodium ions and other ions into nerve cells by preventing the closure of the sodium channels, and not surprisingly the effects of the toxin can be blocked by the administration of tetrodotoxin. The ultimate cause of death is usually cardiac failure, caused by disruption of the balance of sodium and potassium ions.

Of the other toxins produced by frogs of the two genuses, the pumiliotoxins, histrionicotoxins, and gephyrotoxins all act by disrupting ion transport across the membranes of excitable cells. Studies of their various modes of action have contributed greatly to our understanding of neuropharmacology, as well as to helping explain the apparently esoteric alchemical uses of 'eye of newt, and toe of frog'.

Microbial toxins

A much more serious source of human poisoning are the various micro-organisms that contaminate food. So-called paralytic shellfish poisoning is caused by consumption of shellfish that have fed upon certain red algae (dinoflagellates) associated with periodic 'red tides', where massive colonies of these toxic organisms are found. It has been suggested that the first of the ten great plagues of Egypt was caused by such a red tide: '. . . and all the waters that were in the river were turned to blood. And the fish that was in the river died; and the river stank, and the Egyptians could not drink of the water of the river' (Exodus, 7:20, 21). A more recent red tide occurred in the Gulf of Mexico in 1946–7 and left tons of dead fish on the beaches of Florida. The dinoflagellate responsible for this was *Ptychodiscus brevis*, which produces brevetoxins that cause depolarization of nerve and muscle cell membranes, with consequent uncontrolled release of neuro-transmitters. They achieve this by binding to sodium channels and encouraging sodium influx. What is particularly interesting is that the binding site is apparently different from that for tetrodotoxin and saxitoxin (a toxin from a cyanobacterium), which both prevent sodium influx, and from that of batrachotoxin, which enhances sodium influx. Experiments with these neurotoxins are thus revealing much information about the complex structure and functions of the sodium channels.

None of these toxins could be described as genocidal, causing at most hundreds of fatalities per year. More serious contamination of foodstuffs is usually caused by fungi and their constituent mycotoxins. One of the most infamous of these is the fungus *Claviceps purpurea*, which infects rye and other cereals, and was until comparatively recently the biggest killer apart from the bacteria and viruses. The fungus produces ergot alkaloids, which then contaminate rye bread. Certain of these alkaloids produce mainly neurological disturbances in the consumer, and these may be serious enough to initiate convulsions and epileptic seizures. Other alkaloids are vasoconstrictive (they cause narrowing of the blood vessels) and may lead to gangrene of the extremities.

The clinical manifestations of ergotism, as the disease is now known, have been recognized for a long time. As early as 600 BC the Assyrians spoke of 'a noxious pustule in the ear of grain' and the Parsees (in about 350 BC) wrote of 'noxious grasses that cause pregnant women to drop the womb and die in childbed'. But the first well-documented record of ergotism dates from the tenth century and refers to the epidemic of 994 in Aquitaine and Limousin, France. As many as 40 000 people are said to have died: 'Many were tortured and twisted by a contraction of the nerves; others died miserably, their limbs eaten up by the holy fire that blacked like charcoal.' A seventeenth century description of the symptoms is even more vivid:

It seized upon men with a twitching and kind of benumbedness in the hands and feet ... Terrible pains accompanied this evil, and great clamours and screechings did the sick make ... and some had epilepsies, after which fits some lay as it were dead six or eight hours.

The reference to 'holy fire' arose because the people assumed that their blackened (gangrenous) limbs and the burning sensations that they endured were retribution for their sins. Almost inevitably they turned to the Church for help, and in particular prayers were offered to St Anthony, the saint with special powers to protect against fire, infection, and epilepsy. His exemplary life began with a long spell of meditation in the Sinai desert, where he was apparently tortured by visions of licentiousness and weird animals. He survived this ordeal, went on to found Christian monasticism, and died at the age of 105 in AD 356. His remains were brought back from Constantinople in 1070 by returning crusaders and were placed in a church near Vienne in Dauphiné, France. The order of St Anthony was founded in 1093, and the remains became the focus for pilgrimages by those suffering from holy fire. Many miraculous cures were recorded, though these probably owed as much to a change of diet and the attentions of the surgeons at Vienne as they did to the power of prayer; but none the less the power of the Church (and St Anthony) was greatly enhanced.

Ergotism was not only a problem in medieval times. Numerous more recent instances of civil disobedience and episodes of witchcraft have been attributed to the physiological effects of the disease. For example, the alleged bewitchings that occurred in Salem, Massachusetts, in December 1691, may have been caused by a relatively mild outbreak of ergotism. Certainly those affected were said to have been afflicted with various 'distempers' and 'convulsive fits', and during the trials many of the accusers complained that they had suffered much nausea, vomiting, and 'bowels almost pulled out' as a result of being bewitched. Most also complained of hallucinations and 'crawling sensations in the skin'. This last symptom is especially common in victims of ergotism.

A reasonable meteorological record for 1691 is available, and it is clear that the weather pattern was conducive to a good growth of ergot on the local rye, that is, there were early rains and a warm spring followed by a hot, humid summer. In contrast, in 1692 there was a drought, and the

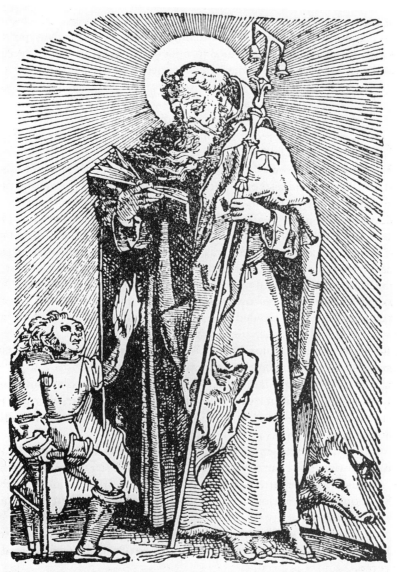

ST. ANTHONY AND A VICTIM OF HIS DISEASE

St Anthony and a victim of ergotism, evidently suffering from the effects of gangrene. Note also that his hand is engulfed with 'holy fire'. (Wellcome Institute Library, London.)

'epidemic of bewitchings' ceased abruptly. We shall obviously never know what caused this 'epidemic of bewitchings', but as a result twenty persons were executed and two more died in prison.

An even more bizarre series of events occurred in France in late July 1789. This has been termed the Great Fear (la Grande Peur), and it involved thousands of peasants in an orgy of destruction mainly directed at the rich landowners. This civil disobedience could, of course, be considered as part of the French Revolution, except that there are numerous records of peasants who had 'lost their heads' (gone insane) and numerous local physicians attributed this to 'bad flour'. The weather conditions in northern France had also been perfect for fungal growth—a moist, warm spring followed by a warm, wet summer. In addition, the peasants were undoubtedly hungry, since the harvest of 1788 had been disastrous, so less care was probably expended on cleaning the rye crop. It is also notable that those areas in which there was no civil unrest had alternative sources of carbohydrate, or had experienced outbreaks of ergotism in the past (as in the Sologne region) and thus took more care in cleaning the crop. Once again we cannot be sure how much ergotism contributed to the surge of peasant unrest that preceded the actual revolution, but its involvement cannot be ignored.

Rye was never a major cereal crop in Britain, but there has been a number of well documented outbreaks of ergotism, such as affected an agricultural labourer's family in Wattisham near Bury St Edmunds in 1762. Two of his children had pains in their legs and the mother and five other children all lost one or both feet or whole legs, though the father only reported numbness in his limbs.

Much more serious epidemics have occurred in Russia during the last three centuries. For example, between September 1926 and August 1927, 11 319 cases were reported out of a population of 506 000 in the vicinity of Sarapoul, which is close to the Urals. However, with a greater awareness of the causes of the disease, ergotism is now extremely rare.

The pharmacology of the ergot alkaloids is clearly of great interest, and their neurological and vasoconstrictive effects will be considered in Chapters 2 and 3 respectively.

Other fungal toxins are more insidious, causing liver or gastrointestinal cancers over a period of many years, though isolated outbreaks of more acute toxicity are also known. The most famous of these toxins are the aflatoxins, which were first identified in 1960 following the deaths of tens of thousands of turkeys in Britain and elsewhere. The birds had consumed peanut meal (from Brazil) contaminated with the fungus *Aspergillus flavus*, and death was due to gross liver damage. There is no direct evidence that liver disease in man can be caused by aflatoxins (although Graham Greene had a character in the *Human Factor* killed by aflatoxin poisoning). However, there is a high incidence of liver cancer in parts of Africa where peanut meal (groundnut meal) is a staple part of the diet. For example, in the highlands of Kenya, where the average daily intake of aflatoxins is 3.5 nanograms per kilogram of body weight per day, the incidence of liver cancer is less than one per 100 000 of the population per year. In parts of Mozambique the corresponding figures are 220 nanograms per kilogram of body weight per day and thirteen cases per 100 000 per year.

Many other mycotoxins have been identified during the last twenty years, mainly produced by strains of *Aspergillus*, *Penicillium*, and *Fusarium*. Most are believed to present a small, though real, long-term hazard to man, and as well as cancer induction their potential for inducing fetal abnormalities (teratogenic effect) is taken most seriously. For example, the aflatoxins are teratogenic if given to rats or hamsters during the middle stages of pregnancy (1–1.5 mg per kilogram of animal weight), but have no effect on mice; their effects on the human fetus are unknown.

Food is most liable to contamination when it is stored under damp conditions, though the optimal temperature for fungal growth varies from species to species: *Aspergillus* prefers temperatures between 20 and 30 °C, while *Fusarium* prefers a temperature in the range 2–15 °C. A dramatic example of the way in which historical circumstances and the weather can affect fungal contamination of food is provided by an episode in Russia during 1942–3. Owing to the prevailing wartime conditions, grain was left in the fields over the winter months and was heavily contaminated with *Fusarium* when harvested. Bread made with this grain caused what became known as alimentary toxic aleukia, characterized by persistent sore throat and a general lowering of the white blood cell count, with associated susceptibility to other infections. Thousands of people died within two weeks of eating the bread.

On a smaller scale, deaths among beer drinkers who have consumed beer made from mouldy grain are not uncommon, and in ancient times this was probably much more prevalent due to contamination of fermenting grain. The toxins present in *Fusarium*-infected products are of the trichothecene family, and these act by inhibiting protein biosynthesis. The trichothecenes achieved star status in the early 1980s when they were reputedly used by the Russians as agents of biological warfare. The Americans claimed that a 'yellow rain' (of *Fusarium* spores) had descended on

Laos, Kampuchea (Cambodia), and Afghanistan, and huge sums of money were devoted to a campaign designed to convince a largely sceptical world of the truth of the allegations.

On 13 September 1981 the Secretary of State, Alexander Haig, announced:

> *For some time now, the international community has been alarmed by continuing reports that the Soviet Union and its allies have been using lethal chemical weapons in Laos, Kampuchea, and Afghanistan ... We now have physical evidence from South-east Asia which has been analysed and found to contain abnormally high levels of three potent mycotoxins—poisonous substances not indigenous to the region and which are highly toxic to man and animals.*

At that stage the physical evidence comprised one leaf and one twig from Kampuchea, both contaminated with trace amounts of trichothecenes, but in due course blood, urine, and other samples were produced from alleged victims to support the case. It should be noted that these persons were mostly illiterate people from the temperate mountains of the countries concerned and would have needed little prompting to accept that they were the victims of chemical warfare.

The main allegations were that trichothecenes did not occur naturally in tropical South-east Asia, or at least not in the amounts isolated. All attempts by independent research workers to substantiate the US claims failed completely. *Fusarium* growths have certainly been observed in tropical and (especially) temperate South-east Asia, so a natural origin for the trichothecenes is entirely reasonable. As to the origin of the 'yellow rain', Charles Darwin reported something similar in 1863, while a 'yellow rainstorm' lasting twenty minutes occurred over an area of twenty acres in China in 1976. Definitive scientific investigations have now shown that the droplets comprise pollen, algae, and other constituents of the faeces of the giant honey-bee *Apis dorsata*. When the beehive is subject to thermal stress, about half of the population of bees fly off and defecate. This ensures a physical loss of heat through the exertions of flying, and in addition the loss of body weight increases the efficiency of body temperature regulation.

So it appears that the alleged chemical warfare was nothing more than a natural phenomenon. The logic behind such an attempt at genocide is flawed anyway, since it has been estimated that about 3 tonnes of pure toxin per square mile would be needed to ensure an effective killing dose. One of the nerve gases would do the job so much more efficiently.

Many other mycotoxins probably contribute to the cause of disease and exacerbate nutritional deficiencies, especially among inhabitants of the developing countries. A literal interpretation of the Old Testament suggests that this has always been the case. Take for example Job's description of his dysentery—'my bowels boiled, and rested not' (Job, 30:27); dermatitis—'my skin is broken, and become loathsome' (7:5); and neurological disturbances—'thou scarest me with dreams, and terrifiest me through visions' (7:14). His circumstances had led him to a state of reliance on (mouldy) vegetables and he suffered the consequences of malnutrition and mycotoxin intoxication.

Even in the developed world mycotoxin contamination is not unknown, and our taste for exotic cheeses and other foods means that we may encounter the mycotoxins produced by *Penicillium roquefortii* and *Penicillium camembertii*, to name but two moulds that are employed in cheese manufacture.

With the exception of these last substances, most mycotoxins are ingested by accident. However, man has always sought edible fungi and many have become an established part of his diet. Of the common fungi, those of the genus *Amanita* are best left alone, because some contain deadly poisons and others produce unpleasant after-effects. As the Swedish mycologist Waldemar Bulow put it: 'They belong to the considerable number of fungi to which it is better to devote pure botanical interest than to give them a place on the table.'

Most deaths in Western Europe and North America that are ascribed to fungal poisoning are caused by the aptly named death cap mushroom, also known as the angel of death, or *Amanita phalloides*. The symptoms of poisoning closely resemble those recorded by many historically famous poison victims, and their delayed onset and the protracted period before death must have been convenient for those wishing to rearrange the victim's financial affairs. About six to twelve hours after consumption of as little as one mushroom (about 50 g), abdominal cramps and vomiting commence, followed by diarrhoea and respiratory distress. Often the symptoms then subside, but after three to eight days liver damage becomes apparent, and death is usually due to liver failure with associated jaundice and coma.

The toxins present in the mushroom are of two types: the phallotoxins and amatoxins. All of these are complex peptides, of which phalloidine and α-amanitine are the most abundant. While the phallotoxins have low mammalian toxicity, the lethal dose for the amatoxins is of the order of 0.1 mg per kilogram of body weight, that is about 5–7 mg for an adult.

However, some good might yet come from α-amanitine, since it specifically inhibits the functions of one of the enzymes involved in the production of RNA, so-called RNA polymerase II. This enzyme is intimately involved with the transcription of the hereditary information present in a cell as DNA into RNA, which is then used as a blueprint for protein production (see Fig. 2.3). The resultant structural proteins (like the collagen of skin and tendon) and catalytically active proteins (enzymes) control our shape, constitution, and biochemistry. α-Amanitine is thus a useful research tool for the investigation of the regulation of RNA and protein production.

Even more infamous than the death cap is the fungus known as fly agaric (*Amanita muscaria*), the red mushroom with white spots beloved of fairy-tale illustrators. It is common in the temperate regions and grows best in damp birchwoods in the autumn, and it has been associated with demons and evil for centuries. In earlier times pulp of the fungus was smeared on to house walls to act as an insecticide, hence the name. But it is the hallucinogenic properties of the fungus which are of most historical interest, and these will be discussed in Chapter 2.

Some mushrooms, though edible, are strictly for teetotallers. One of the more common of these is the common ink cap (*Coprinus atramentarius*). This contains an unusual amino acid, coprine, which inhibits one of the enzymes that is involved in the metabolism of alcohol. When the mushroom is eaten in conjunction with alcohol, the hangover is both immediate and highly unpleasant, involving much nausea and vomiting. In this respect the effects are similar to those experienced with the drug disulfiram (Antabuse), which is used to treat alcoholics, the idea being that unpleasant sensations are then associated with the consumption of alcohol.

Numerous other plants contain toxins that produce unpleasant (though rarely fatal) after-effects, and these are more commonly eaten when more nutritious plants are not available. For example, the root of the cassava plant (*Manihot esculenta*) is an important plant in the tropics and provides the main source of carbohydrate for an estimated 300 million people. It is essentially devoid of protein, being high in starch, and is used to make tapioca. Provided that the fresh root is properly peeled, washed, and cooked, there is no danger, but woe betide the person who cooks the unprepared root in a utensil fitted with a lid, because around 250 mg of hydrogen cyanide can be released from 100 g of fresh root. This is responsible for both acute and chronic cyanide toxicity among cassava users.

Other well known plant products also contain cyanogenic glycosides that release cyanide when the plant tissue is crushed or broken. These

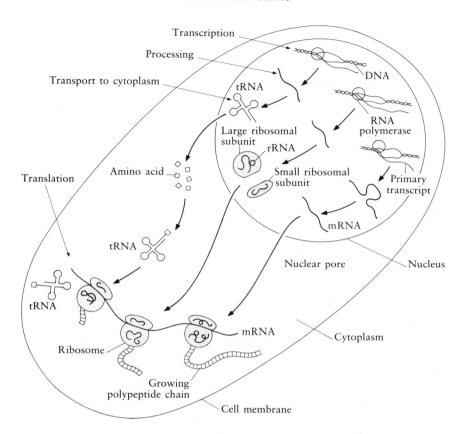

Fig. 2.3 DNA transcription and the biosynthesis of proteins. The process by which genetic information in the form of DNA is used as a blueprint for the production of proteins and enzymes has three states. First, the twin strands of DNA (the double helix) become partially unwound and—with the assistance of the enzyme RNA polymerase—the 'genetic message' is used as a code for the production of RNA. This is transcription. Second, the RNA is processed into a variety of smaller RNA species: transfer RNA (tRNA), messenger RNA (mRNA), and ribosomal RNA (rRNA). These pass out of the nucleus and into the cytoplasm. Here the various kinds of tRNA take up discrete amino acids. These tRNA–amino acid conjugates can recognize signals on mRNA which are specific for the particular type of amino acid. Therefore, as the mRNA threads its way through the ribosome (a complex structure comprising rRNA and a number of different proteins), amino acids are joined together in a prescribed sequence, thus generating a growing polypeptide chain. This ultimately yields the fully formed protein or enzyme. This is translation.

include bitter almonds, the stones of cherries, peaches, and apricots, and immature bamboo shoots. Indeed, extracts from apricot stones have been dispensed under the name of laetrile as a treatment for cancer, though with apparently little efficacy and some premature deaths.

A more dramatic effect is seen with the unripe ackee fruit, *Blighia sapida*, which is common in the West Indies. This produces a dramatic fall in the concentration of blood sugar, especially if children or under-nourished persons consume the unripe fruit, and there is consequent vomiting, convulsions, and even death.

All of these toxins are presumably produced by the fungi or plants for the purpose of deterring passing herbivores and most of them are amazingly effective—who after all would consider the consumption of an ink cap mushroom and alcohol after a prior encounter? However, most deterrents require less esoteric strategies, and man has learned by trial and error which plants and parts of plants are harmful. Take for instance the castor bean (*Ricinus communis*). As mentioned in the Introduction, the expressed oil has useful laxative properties, but the seeds also contain a toxin whose toxicity is only exceeded by the botulinus and tetanus toxins. It is claimed that eight seeds (if chewed) will induce nausea, muscle spasms, vomiting, convulsions, and death. With typical foresight, the US Army took out a patent in 1962 for the use of powdered seeds in chemical warfare.

The toxin is a glycoprotein (a protein with attached carbohydrate chains) called ricin. Part of this complex molecule (the B subunit) functions as an anchor that binds to cells, and the other toxic part of the molecule (the A subunit) then passes into the cell and inhibits the production of protein. This mode of action is currently of considerable clinical interest, because the A subunit is claimed to be more toxic to malignant (cancer) cells than to normal cells. In consequence it has been attached to anti-bodies specific for cancer cells, and when these antibodies home in on the rogue cells they carry with them ricin-A, which then kills the cells. This is a form of drug targeting, and after early clinical trials there is room for guarded optimism for this form of chemotherapy.

Ricin has also been used in a more sinister way, or at least there is good evidence to suggest that the Bulgarian playwright and novelist Georgy Markov was assassinated in London in September 1978 by the Bulgarian secret police using ricin. The toxin was administered using an umbrella with a needle concealed in its tip. With this he was stabbed in the leg, with the result that he died some days later apparently from natural causes.

Such cloak-and-dagger poisoning in the twentieth century can be compared with similar activities described in Shakespeare's plays:

> And, for that purpose, I'll anoint my sword . . .
> . . . that, if I gall him slightly,
> It may be death.
>
> > Hamlet, IV, vii

This chapter will conclude with some examples of poisons that have been widely used by man for nefarious purposes.

Classical poisons II: aconite, arsenic, and hemlock

The plant *Aconitum napellus* is first mentioned in classical mythology. Hercules descended into Hades to capture the three-headed dog Cerberus and, on his return, the dog 'could not stand the rays of the sun, and vomited, and from the vomit sprang the plant . . .' subsequently called *akonitos*, or so claimed Ovid in his *Metamorphoses*. The poisonous nature of the plant was first noted by Hecate, the goddess of witchcraft, who lived with Circe on the island of Colchis. These two were jointly responsible for the introduction of numerous poisons and for the popularization of the art of poisoning.

The plant has had various names since antiquity including wolfsbane (because its root and raw meat were used as bait to kill wolves), monkshood (because the hooded flower resembled a monk's cowl), leopard killer, brute killer, and woman killer. The dried root is the usual source of poison, and this extract was widely used as an arrow poison in many parts of Europe and especially in Asia; but its use by professional poisoners in ancient Rome reached almost epidemic proportions, so much so that cultivation of the plant became a capital offence. However, in the Greek island of Chios its use was sanctioned for euthanasia involving old and infirm men.

The active constituent, aconitine, has been shown to reduce the ion selectivity of sodium channels with a resultant increased uptake of sodium and other ions via these channels. This results ultimately in production of cardiac arrhythmias and depression of respiration. As so often, John Gerard, the Elizabethan herbalist provided one of the the best descriptions of its effects in his *Herball*: 'Their lips and tongs swell forthwith, their eyes hang out, their thighs are stiffe, and their wits are taken from them.'

The symptoms of Napoleon's final illness on St Helena are less extreme, though he is said to have suffered from periodic bouts of nausea and vomiting, diarrhoea, lethargy, muscle weakness, and 'pins and needles' (paraesthesiae). All would be consistent with cancer of the stomach, which

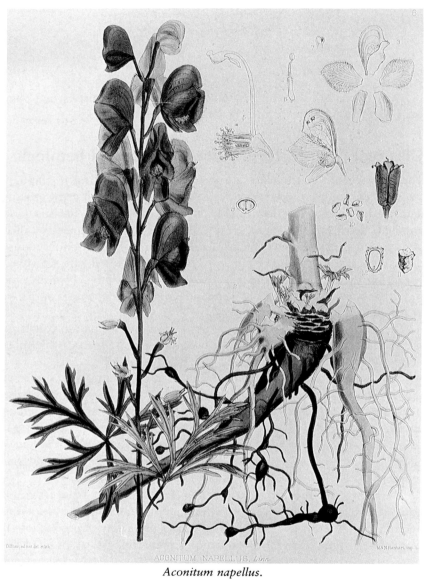

Aconitum napellus.

is the usually accepted condition from which he suffered. However, his death was probably hastened by the administration of a cocktail of the nineteenth century's best medicines. These included tartar emetic (antimony salts), bitter almonds (a source of cyanide), and calomel (mercuric chloride). But most interesting of all is the suggestion that he was also being poisoned with arsenic. Various analyses of available hair samples from Napoleon have demonstrated significant or insignificant levels of arsenic, depending on which authority one believes. As well as a human hand, the source of this arsenic has been ascribed to wallpaper pigments assimilated by moulds which were then released into the air, or to Fowler's solution, which was another therapeutic brew of the time. Whatever the truth, Napoleon seems to have received a veritable witches' brew of toxic metal salts before his death in 1826.

Accidental poisoning with heavy metal salts was especially prevalent following the industrial revolution. Many kinds of new food products contained coloured salts of lead, mercury, copper, and chromium. For example, lead chromate (chrome yellow) was a popular yellow colourant for sweets, custard powder, and snuff, while copper arsenite (Scheele's green) was a constituent of green blancmange and other green confections. The lead present in solder of food cans was another common course of illness and has recently been shown to have been the most likely cause of the deaths of the 129 members of Sir John Franklin's expedition of 1848. During their attempt to discover a north-west sea passage, their ship became trapped in pack-ice, and their subsequent dependence on tinned food, with its lead contaminants, probably dulled their senses and hastened their deaths. The bodies of some members of the expedition were discovered in 1988 and analysis of samples from these remains showed the presence of high levels of lead, consistent with acute lead poisoning.

In the other section on classical poisons, an example of legalized murder (with extract from the upas tree) was presented, and this chapter will end with another, even more famous, example—that of Socrates from hemlock poisoning. The account given by Plato in his *Phaedo* is still moving twenty-three centuries later, and provides a vivid description of the blockade of both sensory and motor neurons, with death ultimately due to respiratory failure:

And the man who gave the poison began to examine his feet and legs . . . then he pressed his foot hard, and asked if there was any feeling in it; and Socrates said No; and then his legs, and so higher and higher, and showed us that he was cold and stiff.

Keats took up the same theme in his 'Ode to a Nightingale':

My heart aches, and a drowsy numbness pains
My sense, as though of hemlock I had drunk.

Other means of altering the senses, through the use of stimulants, hallucinogens, and inebriants will be the subject of the next chapter.

Magic

Mille phantasmata e dæmonu obversatium effigies circumspectarent.

This description of the hallucinogenic effects elicited by the Aztec 'magical' preparation ololiuqui, was recorded by Francisco Hernández, personal physician to Philip II of Spain. He carried out extensive investigations on the flora and fauna of Mexico during the years 1570–75, and his report *Rerum Medicarum Novae Hispaniae Thesaurus* was finally published in 1651. It contains a detailed description of the preparation and use of ololiuqui, and he notes that: 'When the priests wanted to commune with their gods and receive a message from them . . . they ate this plant; and a thousand visions and satanic hallucinations appeared to them.'

This is one of the earliest written accounts of the use of a hallucinogen, and it provides cogent support for the belief that primitive cultures employed psychoactive plant extracts to gain access to the supernatural rather than for pleasure. These aboriginal societies regarded the magical preparations as gifts from the gods, and often deified them. They were used almost exclusively by the priests (or shamans) and were believed to facilitate communication with the spirit world, for the purpose of making diagnosis of disease or predictions of the future. The gods, after all, were thought to control all aspects of human existence: birth, health, fertility, sickness, and death.

Numerous more recent studies have been made of the rituals associated with the collection and use of psychoactive plant extracts, and ethnobotany and ethnopharmacology are now well respected scientific disciplines. Use of such potions was, and still is, largely confined to Central and South America, especially Mexico, though there is no lack of candidate plants in the Old World. This difference is most likely cultural, since the rise of the strong, monotheistic religions, primarily Judaism, Christianity, and Islam, removed the necessity for a belief in the spirit world and for the associated shamanistic rituals.

A totally satisfying classification of the various psychoactive substances is difficult. The German toxicologist and physiologist Lewis Lewin assigned them to five categories: excitantia, inebriantia, hypnotica, euphorica, and phantastica. Albert Hofmann, the discoverer of LSD, described them as stimulants, intoxicants, hypnotics, sedatives and tranquillizers, analgesics and euphoriants, and psychotomimetics and hallucinogens.

In this chapter a simple division into stimulants, psychotomimetics, and inebriants will be used. Thus, opium (which contains mainly morphine), which is an analgesic and euphoriant, will be dealt with in the chapter on medicine. The division is somewhat arbitrary, but it reflects the main ethnopharmacology of the psychoactive substances involved.

Stimulants

In our modern society, mild stimulants like tea and coffee are primarily of social importance, while more potent ones like cocaine and the amphetamines are agents of abuse. In primitive cultures stimulants were valued more for their ability to extend endurance and to alleviate the pangs of hunger than for their social or 'mind-bending' properties. These aboriginal societies must have experimented widely with plant extracts, for there are literally hundreds of well documented native brews, and many of them were of great potency. Administration of the active ingredients was by one of two routes—as a beverage or in the form of a 'quid' to be chewed—and it is convenient to describe the various preparations under these headings.

Beverages

Many stimulant beverages derive their effects from constituent xanthines, such as caffeine, theophylline, and theobromine; and, of these, tea, coffee, cola, cocoa, and maté are probably the best known.

Although Confucius is often credited with the first, albeit oblique, reference to tea in around 500 BC, the first authentic citation is in a dictionary edited by Kuo P'o, which appeared in around AD 350. Tea was a precious commodity in ancient China, and was variously called 'froth of the liquid jade' or more simply *cha*. Bhuddist monks valued it for its supposed medicinal properties and drank it to sustain them through long hours of meditation. The Japanese subsequently adopted many Chinese customs, and the tea ceremony became an integral part of the Zen culture during the fifteenth century. *Cha-no-yu*, or 'the way of tea', is still very much a part of the Japanese way of life, and tea ceremonies can last anything up to four hours, with consumption of a variety of kinds of teas.

The tea plant itself, *Thea sinensis*, now called *Camellia sinensis*, is native to northern Thailand, eastern Burma, Assam, the Yunnan peninsula, and North Vietnam. In consequence, Europeans did not discover tea until the sixteenth century. The first reference to tea appeared in the memoirs of Giovanni Ramusio, published in 1559, entitled *Delle navigationi et viaggi*. The English East India Company first shipped tea in the early part of the seventeenth century, but did not establish its own plantations in India until 1836 and in Ceylon in the 1870s. The Dutch started somewhat earlier and had plantations in Java from 1826. Tea played a small though important part in American history, because the imposition by the British Government of an import duty on tea, and the subsequent civil disobedience by the colonists (the Boston Tea Party, etc.), were a prelude to the War of Independence.

The British are still the largest importers of tea in the world, and there is an annual per capita consumption of about 4.5 kg. The xanthine content of tea is relatively small, and a typical cup of tea might contain around 100 mg of caffeine. This is enough to cause a mild stimulation of the central nervous system. Theophylline is also present in tea. It possesses marked bronchodilator activity. In pure form it has been used in the treatment of asthma.

Just as tea is the drink of the British, coffee is the American social beverage. Americans consume around 8 kg of coffee per person annually, which represents about 250 mg of caffeine per day. The coffee plant, *Coffea arabica*, is probably a native of Ethiopia, and local folklore attributes the discovery of its stimulant properties to a holy man. This cleric wished to stay awake for his meditations, and noting that goats became more frisky if they ate berries from the plant, he prepared a beverage from the berries. Whatever the truth of this tale, coffee cultivation began in earnest, close to the town of Mocha in the Yemen, during the ninth century.

Although the Persian philosopher Avicenna wrote extensively about coffee in the eleventh century, it was unknown in Europe before the sixteenth century. Anthony Sherley introduced *kahveh* into England in

1601, and coffee houses proliferated during that century to support this trade.

South America became a centre of mass cultivation in the eighteenth century, and now the province of São Paulo supplies about one-half of the world's supply of 4.5 million tonnes per annum. Each of the red berries of the coffee plant contains two seeds with a caffeine content of about 1 per cent, and these are dried, aged, and then roasted to produce the familiar coffee beans.

Theobroma cacao is of much greater interest from an ethnopharmacological standpoint, and our knowledge of its aboriginal use derives from the campaign reports of Cortes. In 1519 he invaded the Yucatan peninsula in what is now Mexico, and subjugated the local Mayans. One result of this conquest was a substantial booty which included a ready-made harem of nineteen girls, one of whom could speak the Mayan and Aztec languages. Cortes christened her Doña Marina, and she quickly learnt Spanish so as to serve Cortes as interpreter during the rest of his murderous campaign.

The Aztec kingdom of Montezuma was next to fall, and among the unbelievable wealth Doña Marina revealed to Cortes the secrets of chocolatl. This bitter beverage contained raw cacao beans, red peppers, and various herbs, and was reserved for Montezuma and the Aztec nobility. Doña Marina claimed that this 'food of the gods' had potent aphrodisiac qualities, thus ensuring the success of the chocolatl when it was first introduced into Europe. In 1550 the nuns of Chiapas discovered how to make a primitive cocoa, by dissolving the powdered cacao beans, vanilla, and sugar in water. This refreshing and reputedly aphrodisiac brew became an instant success. By 1700 there were 2000 chocolate houses in London alone. Nowadays most of the beans come from Brazil, Nigeria, and Ghana; and both chocolate and cocoa are derived from beans that have been fermented, roasted, and finally crushed. Theobromine is the major constituent, and this has a similar stimulant effect to that of caffeine, though the 'addictive' nature of chocolate seems to have more to do with the pleasurable effects of its texture and sweetness than with its theobromine content. Chronic consumption of caffeine, in contrast, probably does lead to physical dependency, and the caffeine withdrawal symptoms include headache, fatigue, lethargy, and nervousness.

The other well known stimulant beverages are maté yerba, an infusion of leaves from the South American plant *Ilex paraguayensis*, and cola from seeds of the West African plants *Cola nitida* and *Cola acuminata*. Both have been used for hundreds of years, and the Guarani Indians of Brazil still have tea parties using the greenish infusion of *Ilex* leaves in water, while natives of Jamaica and parts of Africa chew the star-shaped fruits of *Cola nitida* to alleviate the symptoms of hunger and fatigue. The leaves of *Ilex* have a low content of caffeine, but *Cola* seeds have up to 2 per cent of caffeine and are of course the staple of the soft drinks industry.

None of these brews is particularly potent, at least in comparison with the South American brews called guarana and yopa. The former is derived from seeds of the woody liana called *Paullinia cupana*, which is common in the Amazon region. Guarana paste is prepared from crushed seeds, cassava flour, and water, and this paste is then rolled into cylinders and dried. The residue is grated and the resultant shavings are dissolved in hot, sweetened water. Typically the resultant brew contains about 5 per cent caffeine. The explorer Richard Spruce recorded in about 1870 that the Indians of southern Venezuela drank it 'first thing in the morning, on quitting their hammocks, and consider it a preservative against the malignant bilious fevers which are scourge of the region'.

In Colombia, the bark of the related vine, *Paullinia yopa*, contains about 3 per cent caffeine and is used to make yopa. This beverage is claimed to provide the only sustenance for Indians of the Putamayo region, who make a ritual fast each morning.

All of these beverages depend upon xanthines for their stimulant effects, and these arise because the xanthines increase the production of various secondary messengers within the cell (see Introduction). This leads to a general stimulation of numerous biochemical processes and consequent changes in various bodily functions.

Finally, there is one much-used stimulant that does not rely upon xanthines for its effects, and this is qāt, also known variously as gat, chat, tschat, and tschai. This is prepared from young leaves, twigs, and shoots of the African shrub *Catha edulis*, which are either chewed or made into an infusion with hot water. On consumption there is said to be an initial feeling of excitement and gaiety, and even a mild hallucinogenic effect, but the primary result is a general 'boost' and an alleviation of feelings of hunger and fatigue. This is due to the central nervous stimulant effects of norpseudoephedrine, which has a similar structure to the amphetamines. But there is a price to pay, because prolonged use leads to a reduction in the sex drive. This is most clearly evident in the Yemen, where qāt use is prevalent and a high proportion of the men remain bachelors.

Qāt probably originated in Ethiopia, but there is an Arabic reference to it in 1333 and much of the present-day consumption occurs in the Yemen. There is even an apocryphal story that Ethiopian Airlines was founded so that a daily shipment could be ensured. Whatever the truth of this, a similar brew was also invented in North America, and Mormon tea or desert tea were valued for their stimulant properties by settlers and Indians alike. The desert shrub *Ephedra trifurea* was the main component of this infusion, and this too contains norpseudoephedrine as a major constituent.

Quids for chewing

When a quid of plant material is chewed, the constituent stimulants pass straight into the bloodstream via the buccal cavity in the mouth, thus providing an instantaneous 'lift'. It is not surprising, then, that this route of administration is widely used. Three stimulants from three different continents are of prime historical and contemporary importance: betel from Asia, pituri from Australia, and cocaine from South America.

Betel is a concoction made from leaves of the vine *Piper betel* and slices of the seed of the palm *Areca catechu* in admixture with lime, which helps to free the alkaloid constituents from the vegetable matrix. In Asia various spices like cloves, tamarinds, turmeric, and cardamom, are also added to the mix, and the resultant quid is chewed, producing copious amounts of red saliva. An estimated 200 million people in southern Asia and the islands of the Indian and Pacific Oceans use betel at the present time, and although its origins are unknown it has been used for many centuries. It has mild stimulant properties, though some say it produces a feeling of euphoria akin to that produced by alcohol; and, although the constituent alkaloids have been identified, it is not clear how betel exerts its psychoactive effects.

Such uncertainty does not attend the ethnopharmacology of pituri. The Aborigines of Australia have for centuries used the leaves of certain varieties of the desert shrub *Duboisia hopwoodii* as a stimulant. The leaves are roasted, moistened, formed into a quid, then chewed. During social rites known as 'Big Talks', a communal quid was passed around from mouth to mouth. The main constituent, nicotine, increases the production of adrenalin and alleviates feelings of hunger and fatigue, though in large doses it is toxic. As mentioned in the chapter on poisons, the Aborigines used certain varieties of *D. hopwoodii* rich in nornicotine (which is much more toxic than nicotine) to poison water holes in order to stupefy game, or in earlier times to poison the settlers.

Although these plants are of considerable importance, they pale almost into insignificance when viewed alongside the coca plant *Erythroxylon coca* and its active constituent cocaine. The plant was probably first cultivated in central Amazonia, but it is now most extensively cultivated in the foothills of the Andes in Peru and Bolivia. It thrives in the warm, moist

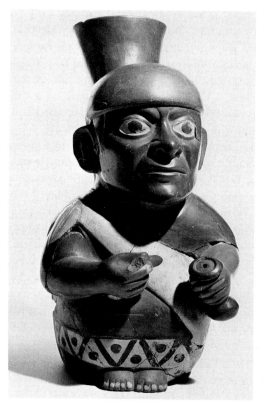

Statuette of a coca user from the Moche III period, c. 300 AD. (From the collection in the Lowie Museum of Anthropology, University of California at Berkeley.)

valleys between 1500 and 6000 metres above sea-level, and the stimulant properties of its leaves have been known from at least the Nazca period (around AD 500). We know this because of the discovery of the mummified remains of a Peruvian potentate of this era accompanied by several bags of coca leaves. In addition, pottery of this period frequently depicts coca chewers with their characteristic distended cheeks.

By the tenth century, when Inca civilization was at its height, coca was well established in the Andes. The Incas believed that the Gods presented coca to the people to satisfy their hunger, to provide them with new vigour, and to help them forget their miseries. They venerated coca and it was intimately involved in their religious ceremonies and in the various initiation rites; and the shamans used it to induce a trance-like state in order to commune with the spirits. It was a far too important commodity to be used by the common Indians, and their exposure to coca was very limited before the invasion by Pizarro and his *conquistadores*.

Pizarro reached the Inca capital, Cuzco, in 1533, and the Inca empire disintegrated in the face of their onslaught. One immediate result was that the Indians could indulge in coca chewing, and cocaine addiction rapidly became prevalent. The Spaniards were impressed with its stimulant properties: 'This herb is so nutritious and invigorating that the Indians labour whole days without anything else.' They capitalized on this, and the Indians were forced to toil in the silver mines with their minds numbed and their appetites suppressed through the consumption of coca.

Coca was first introduced into Europe by the returning *conquistadores*, and wildly exaggerated claims about its properties began to circulate. It was said to be an 'elixir of life', and the *Gentleman's Magazine* in 1814 contained an editorial that exhorted Sir Humphrey Davy (as a leading scientist of the day) to begin experimentation, in the hope that coca could be used as a 'substitute for food, so that people could live a month, now and then, without eating. . .'. But there was no real commercial success before the invention of Vin Mariani. This was the brainchild of Angelo Mariani who introduced his wine, lozenges, and various other preparations in the 1860s. These were claimed to have analgesic, anaesthetic, and carminative properties. They were, not surprisingly, a runaway success given that all of the products contained generous measures of coca extract. Even the Vatican under Pope Leo XIII gave the wine an official seal of approval.

A similar concoction also became popular in the USA under the title of Peruvian Wine of Coca, and an extract from the Sears, Roebuck, and Co. Consumers' Guide of 1900 gives some indication of the wine's attributes:

> *It sustains and refreshes both the body and the brain. . . It may be taken for any length of time with perfect safety . . . it has been effectually proven that in the same space of time more than double the amount of work could be undergone when Peruvian Wine of Coca was used, and positively no fatigue experienced.*

An even more famous beverage, Coca Cola, originally contained extracts of *Erythroxylon coca*, together with extracts of *Cola nitida* (i.e. caffeine), and wine. This was invented by a pharmacist, John S. Pemberton of Atlanta, Georgia. In the early 1880s he introduced a tonic called 'Pemberton's French wine coca'. This was based on Vin Mariani, and Pemberton claimed that it was an excellent tonic, aid to the digestion, and stimulant of the nervous system—an 'intellectual beverage'. When prohibition began in Atlanta in 1886, Pemberton removed the wine from his recipe and replaced it with sugar syrup. He called the new drink 'Coca Cola: the temperance drink'. In 1904 fears about the narcotic properties of

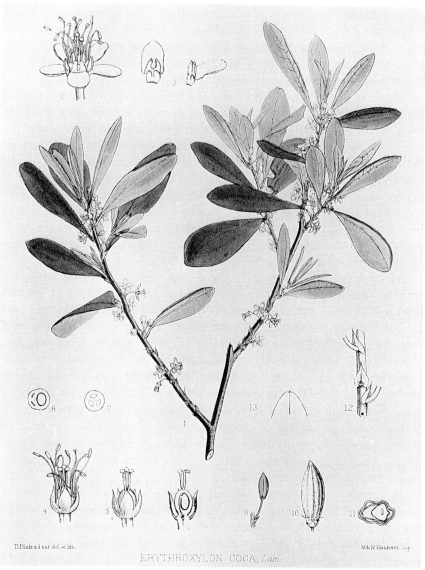

ERYTHROXYLON COCA, *Lam.*

D.Blair, ad nat. del et lith.   M & N Hanhart imp

Erythroxylon coca.

cocaine led to the deletion of the coca extracts, and subsequently the US Government tried to force the Coca Cola Company to change the name of their drink. After much legal wrangling the name was saved, primarily because 'Coca Cola' and 'coke' had become household names, and it was deemed improper for the government to tamper with the language.

Methods for the isolation of cocaine became available in 1860, and Sigmund Freud was one of the first people to experiment with the pure drug. In an enthusiastic report writen in 1884, entitled 'Über Coca', he wrote: 'A few minutes after taking cocaine, one experiences a sudden exhilaration and feeling of lightness. One feels a certain fuzziness on the lips and palate, followed by a feeling of warmth in the same areas.' In a lighter vein, he warned his fiancée Martha Bernays what to expect if he visited her after ingesting cocaine: 'Woe to you my princess when I come. I will kiss you red and feed you until you are plump. And if you are forward, you shall see who is the stronger, a gentle little girl who doesn't eat enough or a big wild man who has cocaine in his body.'

But it was Sigmund Freud's young assistant Carl Köller who first demonstrated the efficacy of cocaine as a local anaesthetic in 1884. He had been asked by Freud to investigate how cocaine alleviated hunger and allayed fatigue, and was experimenting with a dilute solution of the drug in water. He placed some on his tongue, with a resultant numbness and loss of taste. Köller initially investigated the use of cocaine as a local anaesthetic for eye surgery, and after some preliminary animal experiments he and an assistant applied solutions of cocaine to one another's eyes. No sensation was felt when they touched their corneas with a pinhead, and the efficacy of cocaine was established. Köller remained in ophthalmology for many years, first in Vienna, and then in New York; cocaine became the local anaesthetic of choice for the removal of cataracts and for other types of eye surgery.

The mode of action of anaesthetics is still poorly understood, but it is usually stated that cocaine associates with acetylcholine receptors on the nerve membrane and alters the permeability of the membrane to sodium ions, thus interfering with signal transmission. It has now been largely superseded by wholly synthetic drugs like procaine (Novocaine, familiar to all who visit the dentist for treatment), and most of the coca exported from South America is now used for illicit purposes. Absorbed via the mucous membranes in the nose (hence cocaine 'snorting'), it has an immediate and powerful stimulant effect on the pleasure centres of the brain. However, over a period of weeks, it damages the septum in the nose (addicts usually have a runny nose) and also leads to physical dependence.

The addictive properties of cocaine are most marked when the free alkaloid is smoked. This is the currently infamous 'crack', which provides what addicts often describe as 'an orgasm in every cell of one's body'. There is an intense 'high' followed very rapidly by profound depression and a craving for more cocaine. Addicts will smoke crack at fifteen minute intervals for anything up to seventy-two hours, without eating or sleeping, and then simply collapse (or 'crash').

Some understanding of the pharmacology of this addiction is now available, and it seems that cocaine blocks the re-uptake of the neurotransmitter dopamine in the brain. This substance is especially important in those parts of the brain which control pleasure responses, the so-called pleasure centres; and like other synapses, those involving dopamine have a salvage mechanism for unused neurotransmitter. By blocking the uptake of excess dopamine, cocaine potentiates its effects on the pleasure centre neurons (see Fig. 3.1).

In 1988 the National Institute for Drug Abuse estimated that 35–40 million Americans had tried cocaine in one form or another, and the habit

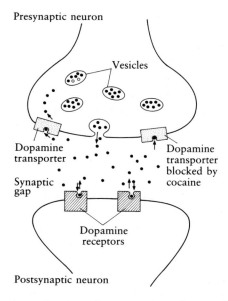

Fig. 3.1 Mechanism of action of cocaine. Stimulation of a dopaminergic nerve terminal causes dopamine to be released from vesicles; it then crosses the synaptic gap and acts on dopamine receptors on the postsynaptic neuron. Cocaine blocks the re-uptake of excess dopamine, which therefore floods the synapse.

is now also a problem in most other parts of the world. In contrast, in South America it is still widely chewed, and it is usually reckoned that at least 15 million Indians are habitual users of coca, the so-called *coqueros*. They use it to increase endurance, to suppress hunger, to impart a feeling of well-being, but probably most importantly to alleviate the misery of their daily lives. The mechanism of action of cocaine is here similar to, though quite distinct from, that involved in the brain. At adrenergic neural junctions the excess of the transmitter noradrenalin is taken up into the releasing or receiving cells, and is then not available to interact with noradrenalin receptors. Cocaine inhibits this re-uptake and thus potentiates the activity of the transmitter, with resultant effects on endurance, etc.

The Indians prepare their quids from coca leaves and a little lime, which interacts with the cocaine salts present in the leaves to liberate the free drug, and the average daily intake of cocaine via this route is likely to be around 400 mg from around 50 g of leaves. This is a similar figure to the amount of cocaine absorbed by a typical 'snorter', but the Indians may actually obtain some benefit from the leaves. These are high in vitamins C, B1, and riboflavin, and chewing quids may help to prevent scurvy and other deficiency diseases in regions where fresh fruit and vegetables are in short supply. The Indians also use coca to relieve the pains of rheumatism and headache, as an aphrodisiac, and to relieve the symptoms of asthma. However, there is little evidence of efficacy.

At the present time we can thus view at least 1500 years of Indian culture based upon coca, about 100 years of clinical utility, and perhaps ten to fifteen years of serious drug abuse, all dependent upon the same stimulant, cocaine.

Psychotomimetics

Old World psychotropic plants and fungi

The stimulant effects of the plants just described were the main reason for their use; their 'mind-bending' properties, where these exist, were incidental. In contrast, the plants and fungi that contain hallucinogenic substances were prized for their magical properties. It must have been a truly 'mind-blowing' experience for the primitives who first experimented with ololiuqui or the fly agaric mushroom, and their aboriginal societies quite understandably revered this new and astounding magic.

To define what constitutes a hallucination or to clearly identify a pure hallucinogen is not easy. Hoffer and Osmond in a book entitled *Hallucinogens* described hallucinogens as:

Chemicals which, in non-toxic doses, produce changes in perception, in thought and in mood, but which seldom produce mental confusion, memory loss, or disorientation for person, place and time.

And this is more or less a restatement of Albert Hofmann's classical description:

In a specific manner [hallucinogens] elicit profound psychic changes associated with changes in perception of reality of space and time . . . body image and personality. Nevertheless consciousness is retained.

In other words, they produce an altered state of consciousness, a kind of dream world, in which the user experiences vastly altered perceptions of space, time, colour, sound, touch, smell, and taste; yet there is no clouding of the senses as there is with alcohol or morphine. It is immediately apparent why the shamans generally kept their secret to themselves, or at most shared their magical preparations with an apprentice or with a patient undergoing diagnosis for disease.

The use of hallucinogenic plants was most highly developed in the New World, especially in Central and South America, and these plants are still widely used. But there were several Old World plant extracts that were of great ethnopharmacological significance: soma, hashish, and the various witches' brews.

Soma

In Aldous Huxley's *Brave New World* soma was the social drug of the future. It had 'all the avantages of Christianity and alcohol; none of their defects' and it allowed the people to 'take a holiday from reality whenever you like, and come back without so much as a headache or a mythology'.

There is no question that the name originates from Soma, the moon god of ancient India, and was used to describe an intoxicating beverage obtained from a sacred plant. The actual identity of this plant is in doubt, even though soma is mentioned in around 150 hymns of the Rig-Veda. This contains writings in Sanskrit of the early Aryan inhabitants of the Indus basin. These Aryans are believed to have invaded India from what is now Afghanistan, and the Rig-Veda is thought to have been written between 1500 and 500 BC. The plant is variously described as having pendant branches and fleshy stalks and to be of a reddish tint. The 'fragrant liquor' obtained by squeezing the stalks was said to produce intoxication and a feeling of strength and courage. It also possessed aphrodisiac properties. Soma was very much a holy brew and was itself worshipped.

Various plants have been suggested as the soma of Vedic India, and various milkweeds, such as *Sarcostemma acidum* and *Sarcostemma brevis-tigma*, are used in present-day India to provide extracts known as soma. *Cannabis sativa*, from which hashish and marijuana are obtained, was also once believed to be the soma of ancient India. However, it is now widely accepted that the mushroom *Amanita muscaria* was the most likely source of soma.

Amanita muscaria is the familiar red mushroom with white spots often illustrated in books of children's fairy tales, and it is widespread in the temperate parts of the northern hemisphere. It grows particularly well under fir and birch trees and is a common sight on damp, autumnal days. As mentioned in the chapter on poisons, it was originally valued as an insecticide, hence the name fly agaric, but its use as a source of hallucinogens in parts of north-eastern Asia and Siberia is also ancient. Most of our information about the magical properties of this mushroom comes from a scholarly work by R. G. Wasson, entitled *Soma the Divine Mushroom*. He studied the translations of the Rig-Veda and also collated all of the accounts of Asian and Scandinavian explorers who had encountered fly agaric use. He concluded that the soma of ancient India and fly agaric were one and the same. In particular, he identified various phrases in the Vedic hymns that seem to describe *Amanita muscaria*, with its characteristic shape and rosy red hue with white projections. For example: 'by day he [the mushroom] appears *hari* [colour of fire], by night silvery white' and 'soma with his thousand knobs [or studs]'. The book is full of learned speculation, but whatever the source of soma, Wasson also provided a fascinating collection of travellers' tales about fly agaric. Probably the earliest description by a European of mushroom consumption was the account given by Filip von Strahlenberg, a Swedish colonel, who was held for twelve years as a prisoner of war by the Koryak tribe in north-eastern Siberia and returned to publish his memoirs in 1730. He records:

> *Those who are rich among them, lay up large provisions of these mushrooms, for the winter. When they make a feast, they pour water upon some of the mushrooms, and boil them. They then drink the liquor, which intoxicates them. The poorer sort . . . post themselves, on these occasions, round the huts of the rich, and watch the opportunity of the guests coming down to make water; and then hold a wooden bowl to receive the urine, which they drink off greedily . . ., and by this way they also get drunk.*

A similar account was provided by Georg Steller, who spent several years with the Koryak, and wrote in 1774:

The fly agarics are dried, then eaten in large pieces without chewing them, washing them down with cold water. After about half an hour the person becomes completely intoxicated and experiences extra-ordinary visions. Those who cannot afford the fairly high price [of the mushrooms] drink the urine of those who have eaten it, where-upon they become as intoxicated, if not more so. The urine seems to be more powerful than the mushroom, and its effect may last through the fourth or fifth man.

Many of the accounts describe the hallucinogenic effects of the mushroom, and they mostly agree that about an hour after ingestion there is a period of mild euphoria accompanied by pseudo-religious visions. The account by Stephan Krasheninnikov, published in 1755, and with a fresh translation by Wasson, states: 'They are subject to various visions, terrify-ing or felicitous ... owing to which some jump, some dance, others cry and suffer great terrors, while some might deem a small crack to be as wide as a door, and a tub of water as deep as the sea.'

A more familiar description of what may be fly agaric intoxication was written by Lewis Carroll in *Through the Looking Glass*:

'Come, my head's free at last!' said Alice in a tone of delight, which changed into alarm in another moment, when she found that her shoulders were nowhere to be found: all she could see, when she looked down, was an immense length of neck, which seemed to rise like a stalk out of a sea of green leaves that lay far below her.

Certainly Lewis Carroll was familiar with Cooke's *Manual of British Fungi*, which was the main source of information available at the time, but his description of the effects of a hallucinogen is so accurate that it is tempting to speculate that he may have experienced the effects himself.

The use of this mushroom is still widespread in various parts of Siberia among the Finno-Ugrian peoples, the Ostyak and the Vogul, and among the Chukchi, Koryak, and Kamchadal peoples. In former times it may have been the source of hallucinogen for the Norse berserkers, though a more reasonable source seems to be the related species *Amanita pantherina*, which is known to produce mania if ingested, though the active ingredient is not known. The psychoactive constituents of fly agaric are thought to be muscimol and ibotenic acid, though the mushroom also contains muscarine. This latter compound is of particular historical importance, because as early as 1869 Schmiedeberg demonstrated that muscarine could elicit excitation of the vagus nerve in frogs. This stimulated the search for neurotransmitter substances that led ultimately to the discovery of acetyl-choline. Muscarine can mimic the effects of acetylcholine at parasympathetic nerve-endings by interacting with one subclass of acetylcholine receptors, the muscarinic receptors.

Ibotenic acid and muscimol probably exert their pharmacological effects through interference with the normal functioning of the brain neurotransmitter γ-aminobutyric acid (GABA). This is an inhibitory neurotransmitter, which is active at up to 40 per cent of brain synapses. It appears to function (at least in part) by opening channels in the neuronal membrane specific for chloride ions. This makes the inside of the cell more negative, so that many more sodium ions must enter before depolarization can occur. The two mushroom alkaloids presumably bind to GABA receptors in the channel and block the inrush of chloride ions, thus preventing the inhibition of brain activity caused by GABA. A comparison of the structures of ibotenic acid, muscimol, and GABA is shown in Fig. 3.2.

The GABA-dependent neuronal systems have been much studied, since in addition to these interactions with muscimol and ibotenic acid there are also interactions with the benzodiazepine tranquillizers such as Valium.

As to the pharmacology of the urine of mushroom users, no research seems to have been conducted, but it is possible that ibotenic acid is decarboxylated (loses carbon dioxide) to yield the more potent muscimol as it passes through the body.

Hashish

While the origin of soma is lost in the mists of time, the history of hashish is well documented. As early as 2000 BC, in the reign of the legendary emperor Shen-Nung, it was written that 'hemp fruit' would result in the users 'seeing devils' (having hallucinations), though communication with less malevolent spirits was the probable intention. The wild Scythian horsemen inhaled the smoke from burning hemp seeds, or so claims Herodotus, who wrote in about 500 BC: 'A dish is placed on the ground into which they put a number of red hot stones and then add some hemp seed . . . immediately it smokes and gives out such a vapour . . . the Scyths, delighted, shout for joy.' Recent archaeological evidence seems to support the reality of this practice. By AD 200 the Greek physician Galen was able to report the widespread use of hemp in cakes, etc., to produce hilarity and enjoyment at dinner parties.

But to stress the importance of the psychoactive properties of the plant *Cannabis sativa* in this historical context would be misleading. The plant almost certainly originated in central Asia, and was initially valued for its

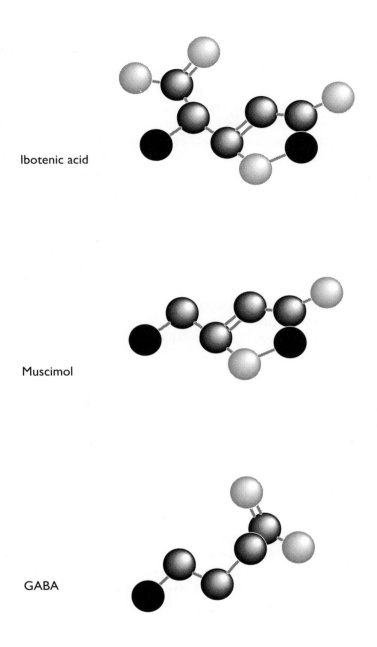

Ibotenic acid

Muscimol

GABA

Fig. 3.2 Comparisons of the structures of ibotenic acid, muscimol, and GABA.

strong fibrous stem. Traces of hemp rope dating from about 3000 BC have been found in Turkestan, and it is likely that a limited amount of selective breeding was undertaken to improve this property of the plant. The seeds were also important as a source of protein and for their oil, which was used to light lamps in biblical times.

Rope manufacture remained the major use for hemp until quite recently, and certainly the evolution of the British navy under Henry VIII in the fifteenth century and its supremacy until well into the twentieth century, depended upon a good supply of hempen rope. *Cannabis sativa* was cultivated as a fibre plant in Roman Gaul and probably in Roman Britain as well, and it was well established in Britain by the time of the Norman conquest (1066). The plant was exported to Canada (1606), Virginia (1611), and New England (1632) by British colonists, and was quite separately introduced into South America in the mid-sixteenth century by Spanish adventurers.

Its medicinal properties were also valued, and the Emperor Shen-Nung mentioned its use as a treatment for malaria, beri-beri, rheumatic pains, etc., while Indian medicine claimed that it was useful in the treatment of leprosy, venereal disease, mania, and less serious conditions like dandruff and insomnia. In Europe the medieval physicians perpetuated the prescriptions and remedies introduced by Galen and Dioscorides, and they distinguished between natural hemp ('bastard hempe') for the treatment of 'nodes and wennes and other hard tumours' and cultivated hemp ('manured hempe') for less serious conditions. Not surprisingly, its psychoactive properties were often of value in these medicines, and various analgesic concoctions were used. To this day, women in Lesotho smoke cannabis as part of their preparations for childbirth.

Returning to its use as a hallucinogen, it is Indian culture that provides much of our information about the use of *Cannabis* before the thirteenth century. Just as with soma, the crude extract of the plant, usually referred to as 'bhang', was revered. The name 'bhang' is now applied to a preparation made from the pulverized green leaves, mixed with milk or water or compounded with spices, and it is likely that the 'sacred nectar' of Vedic India was something similar. The Hindu god Shiva insisted that the word *bhangi* should be chanted by those involved in any part of the cultivation of the plant, and other similar superstitions abound in the mythology of ancient India.

Marco Polo is usually credited with the first European account of hemp consumption. In the report of his travels in the late-thirteenth century, he described the exotic and barbarous practices of the sect established by the

Persian warlord known as Al-Hasan ibn al-Sabbah or Alaodin or simply the Old Man of the Mountain (*Il Veglio della Montagna*). This Mohammedan sect, known as the Assassins (*Assassini*), were fanatical political terrorists whose stated aim it was to rid the Muslim world of false prophets. They were totally fearless and seemed to accept their almost inevitable capture, torture, and death as a form of reward.

This amazing behaviour was assumed to be due to the influence of some kind of potion administered by Alaodin and his successors, and the folk-belief was that hemp was involved. An artificial paradise had supposedly been created in Alaodin's mountain fortress, complete with a beautiful garden, fair damsels, and four fountains that provided wine, milk, honey, or water. Young recruits were drugged, and when they awoke they believed themselves to be in Paradise, or were told that it was at least a foretaste of Paradise. When called upon to make the supreme sacrifice, they went gladly to their deaths. Or so Marco Polo would have us believe.

There is no evidence that Marco Polo ever approached the Old Man's stronghold, which was in the Persian province of Mazandaran, to the south of the Caspian Sea, not far from what is now Teheran. The Assassins certainly existed, and had been feared throughout Europe and Asia since the twelfth century. The etymology of the word 'assassin' is also well-established: it derived from the Arabic word *ḥashshāshīn* meaning 'hashish eaters'. Hashish is a preparation made from the resin of the flowering tops of *Cannabis sativa*, and it is one of the more potent psychoactive forms of the hemp plant. It is claimed that use of the plant began in Persia as early as the sixth century AD, and hashish eating is still widely practised in Arab countries. However, none of the authoritative Mohammedan accounts of the Assassins ever mentioned their use of hashish, and this is surprising, because it would have helped to discredit what was a pseudo-religious sect.

The pharmacology is also suspect. Marco Polo states that the volunteer Assassins were given drinks which made them sleep—'li fa loro dare beveraggio che dormono'; and then they were carried into the garden with the wondrous fountains, etc., so that when they awoke they believed they were in Paradise: 'Quando color si svegliono, trovansi quivi, molto si maravigliano, e sono molto tristi che si truovano fuori del paradiso.'

Hashish is not usually sleep-inducing, and it produces a dreamy state with a heightened perception of sound and colour, so something more potent (and narcotic) must have been part of the induction brew. It is also doubtful whether fighting men could have stayed in the peak of condition on a diet of drugs, drink, and sex. None the less, despite these pharmacological discrepancies and possible etymological problems, there is no doubt that Marco Polo's report of his travels brought hashish to the attention of the European nations, and the word 'assassin' entered the dictionaries.

Cannabis was not widely used in Europe until after Napoleon's campaigns in the Middle East. His soldiers, and also British doctors returning from tours of duty in India, introduced the plant and the habit. Consumption of hemp products in Europe reached a kind of cultural apogee in the nineteenth century, when French writers formed a select club known as 'Le club des Hashishins'. Prominent among its members were the poets Charles Baudelaire, Honoré de Balzac, and Théophile Gautier, and most of them wrote accounts of their use of hashish to improve artistic performance. Baudelaire, for example, recorded the results of his experiments with hashish, wine, and opium in his book *Les paradis artificiels*. Consumption of the drug in the right circumstances ('vous avez eu la précaution de bien choisir votre moment pour cette aventureuse expedition') produced distortions of time and space ('les proportions du temps et de l'être sont complètement dérangés par la multitude et l'intensité des sensations et des idées') and a feeling of good humour and tranquillity ('je me trouvais dans un état de langueur et d'étonnement qui était presque du bonheur').

In the same book, Gautier described the heightened awareness of sight and sound: 'Les sens deviennent d'une finesse et d'une acuité extraordinaire. Les yeux percent l'infinii. L'oreille perçoit les sons les plus insaisissables au milieu des bruits les plus aigus.' And more poetically: 'Les sons ont une couleur, les couleurs ont une musique. Les notes musicales sont des nombres, et vous résolvez avec une rapidité effrayante de prodigieux calculs d'arithmetique.'

Another Frenchman, the psychiatrist Moreau, experimented with hashish and various other psychoactive substances in a more scientific way, and also studied the folk use of the drug in Egypt and the Middle East. He concluded that hashish contained a substance which produced mental states resembling those associated with various psychoses. In his book *Du hachisch et de L'aliénation mentale* he provided the first (pseudo-)scientific classification of the effects of hashish. He divided these into eight categories: euphoria, loss of concentration, distortion of time and space, enhanced aural acuity, illusions, emotional excitement, impulsiveness, and hallucinations.

In reality it is probably doubtful whether the various forms of hemp produce anything other than mild euphoria (at least in moderate doses), and the main danger associated with its consumption is that it brings the consumer into proximity with the suppliers of more dangerous drugs. It is certainly used in its various forms by vast numbers of people. In the Far East, especially in India, three forms of *Cannabis* are employed: the relatively weak bhang and two strong, resinous preparations called ganja and charas, which are obtained from the flowering tops of selected, wild 'races' of the plant. In the Middle East hashish is predominant, while in Africa the leaves are dried and then smoked, usually in conjunction with tobacco. In the past the natives simply inhaled the smoke from heaps of smouldering hemp.

The smoking of marijuana was introduced into the USA as recently as the 1920s by immigrant Mexican workers, and the practice is now widespread. 'Smoking pot' is in fact legal in many states, e.g. California, but is a criminal offence in many others.

Much work has been done on the pharmacology of *Cannabis sativa*, and there is no doubt that the main psychoactive constituent is Δ^1-tetrahydrocannabinol (THC). However, although its myriad biological effects have been ascribed to changes in the concentrations of catecholamines (adrenalin and noradrenalin) and of serotonin, no definitive explanation of its pharmacology has been given. It has been estimated that to produce a euphoric state, something of the order of 25–50 μg (micrograms) per kilogram of body weight of THC must be taken in via the lungs, or 50–200 μg per kilogram via the gastrointestinal tract. The corresponding hallucinogenic doses are 200–250 μg per kilogram (lungs) and 300–500 μg per kilogram (gastrointestinal tract). In the USA the consumption of one or two 'joints' per day is commonplace, and this corresponds to about 5–10 mg of THC. An Indian ganja user might take in 30–60 mg of THC from 1–2 g of hemp. The social user in the USA should thus experience mild euphoria, while the Indian uses a hallucinogenic dose. Numerous clinical evaluations have also been executed, and, although Δ^1-tetrahydrocannabinol and various synthetic analogues have shown some promise in the treatment of asthma (it causes dilation of the bronchioles), epilepsy (it reduces the number of convulsive episodes), anorexia (it stimulates the appetite), and the sickness induced by cancer chemotherapy, no serious clinical utility has been identified, except for the last condition.

The cytotoxic (cell-killing) drugs employed in the treatment of cancer almost invariably induce vomiting, and this is sometimes so debilitating that the patient refuses further courses of the potentially life-saving drugs. There are, of course, many synthetic anti-emetic agents available, but the discovery that marijuana had this property was intriguing. It is also part of modern folklore.

In the mid-sixties stories began to circulate within the hippy culture that consumption of alcohol and marijuana at parties less often led to sickness than consumption of alcohol alone. But one of the first reports of *Cannabis sativa* in a clinical setting was provided by the American poet Ted Rosenthal in his book *How Could I Not Be Among You?* In this he describes his fight against leukaemia, to which he finally succumbed in 1972:

> *Asparaginase, the drug that I have been on for the last couple of weeks causes acute nausea that no drug, no pill will do anything to help. So my doctors came rushing in one day . . . and said, 'Do you have any weed . . . grass, pot, marijuana?' So I got some that night and I sat there and I decided to wait until I thought I was at my worst. I sat there with a bowl in my lap, ready to vomit and a pipe of pot in my other hand. And just when I was about to let loose, I took a puff and, whee, it was gone. I felt fine. I went right in after two or three puffs and I ate a dozen crabs and a huge lobster and piece of chocolate cake on top of that.*

The pharmaceutical industry was already heavily involved in making and testing analogues of THC for a whole range of pharmacological effects, so it was relatively easy to screen THC and these analogues for anti-emetic activity. In 1982 the American company Eli Lilly announced that one analogue in particular, which they called nabilone, was particularly effective for the prevention of sickness associated with cancer chemotherapy and it has since been widely used for this purpose.

So after five thousand years of use, the hemp plant is still widely prized and used mainly for its psychotropic properties. In contrast, it is very likely that future research will lead to THC analogues that are valued because they combine clinical utility with a lack of unwanted psychotropic effects.

Witches' brew

Of all the plant species used by man, few have as many associations with murder, magic, and medicine as the trio *Atropa belladonna*, *Hyoscyamus niger*, and *Mandragora officinarum*. The use of deadly nightshade, henbane, and mandrake as sources of poisons has already been mentioned in Chapter 1, but they also have a long association with soothsaying, magic, and witchcraft.

In ancient Greece it was believed that people under the influence of henbane became prophetic, and the priestesses of the Delphic oracle are claimed to have inhaled the smoke from smouldering henbane. In Roman times wine adulterated with deadly nightshade was probably consumed

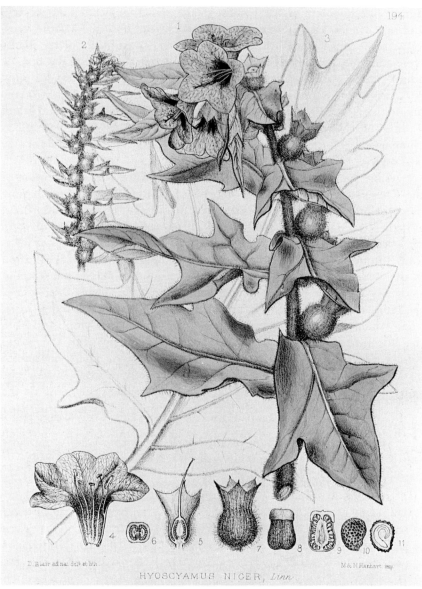

Hyoscymus niger.

during Bacchanalian orgies, but use of the plants for witchcraft, sorcery, and other nefarious activities was not widespread until the Middle Ages.

At some stage it was discovered that if the constituents of the plants were combined with fats or oils they would penetrate through the skin, or could be easily asborbed via the sweat ducts (e.g. in the armpits) or body orifices (e.g. the vagina and rectum). This allowed the psychoactive tropane alkaloids, especially hyoscine, to gain access to the bloodstream and brain, without passage through the gut, with the attendant risks of poisoning. A comparison of the structures of the tropane alkaloids hyoscine and cocaine is shown in Fig. 3.3.

Despite suggestions that the menace of witchcraft was an invention of the Church, used to encourage good Christian behaviour, there is now overwhelming evidence that a variety of strange activities did occur. Whether the participants practised devil worship or not, many of them experienced hallucinations induced by the consumption of tropane alkaloids. Numerous reports contain statements about the mode of application of the 'witches' salves' or 'oyntments'. For example, in an investigation of Lady Alice Kyteler in 1324, the inquisitors stated: 'In rifleing the closet of the ladie, they found a pipe of oynment, wherewith she greased a staffe, upon which she ambled and galloped through thick and thin.' And from the fifteenth century records of Jordanes de Bergamo: 'But the vulgar believe, and the witches confess, that on certain days or nights they anoint a staff and ride on it to the appointed place or anoint themselves under the arms and in other hairy places.' It also explains why so many of the pictures of the time depict partially clothed (or naked) witches astride their broomsticks.

A very detailed description of an experiment with a witch's ointment was provided by Anres Laguna, physician to Pope Julius III, in 1545:

> *. . . a jar half-filled with a certain green unguent . . . with which they were anointing themselves . . . was composed of herbs . . . which are hemlock, nightshade, henbane, and mandrake: of which unguent . . . I managed to obtain a good canister-full . . . which I used to anoint from head-to-toe the wife of the hangman (as a remedy for her insomnia). On being anointed, she suddenly slept such a profound sleep, with her eyes open like a rabbit (she also fittingly looked like a boiled hare), that I could not imagine how to wake her.*

Despite all their efforts, she could not be aroused until thirty-six hours later, whereupon she exclaimed: 'Why do you wake me at such an inopportune time? I was surrounded by all the pleasures and delights of the world.'

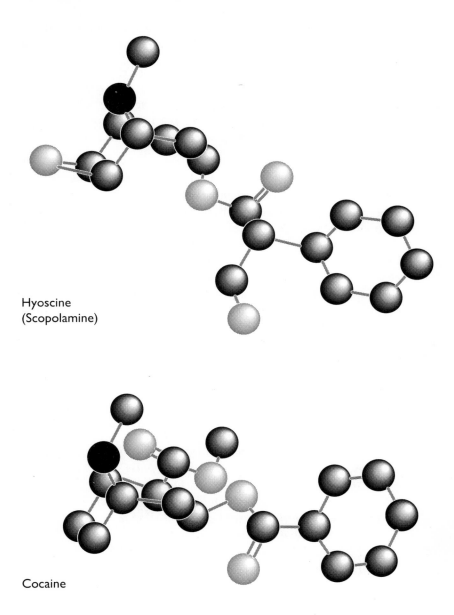

Hyoscine
(Scopolamine)

Cocaine

Fig. 3.3 Comparison of the structures of hyoscine and cocaine.

These 'pleasures and delights' usually involved vivid episodes of flying and orgiastic adventures, as described in the report by Porta, a friend of Galileo:

Thus, on some moonlit night they think that they are carried off to banquets, music, dances, and coupling with young men, which they desire the most. So great is the force of the imagination and the appearance of the images, that the part of the brain called memory is almost full of this sort of thing.

Such accounts have often been ascribed to the effects of the tortures inflicted by the inquisitors; and certainly the men of the Inquisition would not have been above putting words into the mouths of victims on the rack, in order to extract a quick confession. But there are twentieth century accounts of the hallucinogenic effects of witches' salves, such as the report by Will-Erich Peukart, who made a flying ointment based upon a seventeenth century formulation involving use of deadly nightshade, henbane, and *Datura* species. He and some colleagues rubbed ointment on their foreheads and armpits, and then fell into a deep sleep, during which they dreamt of 'wild rides' and 'frenzied dancing'. The death-like sleep induced by *Atropa belladonna* was mentioned by the great Elizabethan herbalist Gerard: 'This kind of Nightshade causeth sleepe ... it bringeth such as have eaten thereof into a dead sleepe wherein many have died.' This semi-comatose state was also familiar to Shakespeare. Take, for example, the account of the effects of the potion given to Juliet by Friar Laurence:

And this distilled liquor drink thou off;
When presently through all thy veins shall run
A cold and drowsy humour, for no pulse
Shall keep his native progress, but surcease;
No warmth, no breath, shall testify thou liv'st;
The roses in thy lips and cheeks shall fade
To paly ashes; thy eyes' windows fall,
Like death, when he shuts up the day of life;
Each part, depriv'd of supple government,
Shall, stiff and stark and cold, appear like death;
And in this borrow'd likeness of shrunk death
Thou shalt continue two-and-forty hours,
And then awake as from a pleasant sleep.
Romeo and Juliet, IV, i

But the most graphic description of tropane alkaloid intoxication was

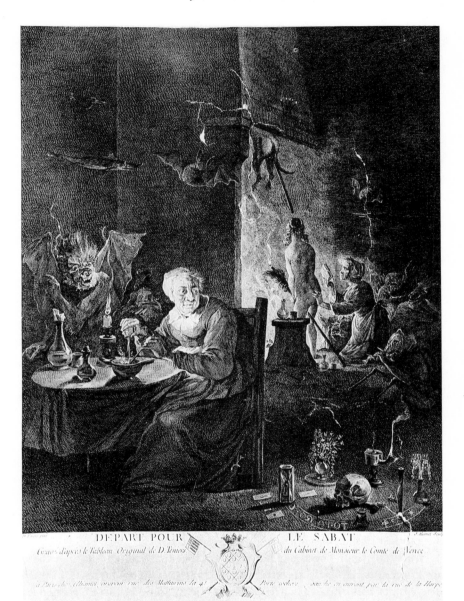

DEPART POUR LE SABAT

An eighteenth century engraving of a witch being prepared for the Sabbat.
Note the administration of the salve. (Wellcome Institute Library, London.)

given by Gustav Schenk in 1966, who inhaled smoke from burning henbane seed:

My teeth were clenched, and a dizzy rage took possession of me . . . but I also know that I was permeated by a peculiar sense of well-being connected with the crazy sensation that my feet were growing lighter, expanding and breaking loose from my body. Each part of my body seemed to be going off on its own, and I was seized with the fear that I was falling apart. At the same time I experienced an intoxicating sensation of flying . . . I soared where my hallucinations —the clouds, the lowering sky, herds of beasts, falling leaves . . . billowing streamers of steam and rivers of molten metal—were swirling along.

There is thus little doubt that the witches did indeed experience 'flights of fancy', primarily due to the effects of hyoscine. Whether the consumer believed that they had been turned into an animal (most commonly a wolf as in lycanthropy), or simply experienced flying and frenzied dancing, probably depended upon the actual brew and the dose of hyoscine. This is known to induce intoxication, followed by a transition from consciousness to narcosis, during which vivid hallucinations often occur. It exerts this depressant activity through an inhibition of the muscarinic subclass of acetylcholine receptors in the central nervous system. Interestingly, all of the tropane alkaloids also prevent secretion from glands that are inner-vated by acetylcholine. In particular, the flow of saliva and of mucus in the respiratory tract is much reduced, and this is one of the non-hallucinogenic side effects reported by both witches and werewolves.

The euphoriant and antisecretory effects of hyoscine are exploited when the drug is used as a premedication before surgery. It also has anti-emetic activity (prevents sickness) and can pass through the skin into the bloodstream (trans-dermal delivery) if coated on to a plaster (Band-Aid). American astronauts have used these hyoscine plasters as a treatment for the motion sickness experienced during space travel.

We shall never know exactly what occurred at Sabbats, though there are numerous scholarly accounts that include eyewitness reports of satan-istic rituals and orgiastic activities, but at least some of these experiences were more in the mind than actual physical reality.

Datura

Hyoscine is also a major constituent of many species of *Datura*. Not only does this genus have a long association with magic and medicine, but also the discovery of its hallucinogenic and medicinal potential occurred independently in both the Old World and the New World. In the former *Datura* was mainly prized for its medicinal properties, but in the latter it has been associated primarily with magico-religious activities.

The name of the genus appears in early Sanskrit writings as *dustura*, and Avicenna, the eleventh century Persian physician, refers to the medicinal and hallucinogenic properties of *datora* or *tatora*. In Asia *Datura metel* and *Datura fastuosa* were widely employed for the treatment of just about every medical condition, including fevers, mental disorders, heart disease, and pneumonia, probably with little efficacy. However, the plants were also combined with *Cannabis* and wine to produce a useful anaesthetic for surgical operations. The hallucinogenic potential of hyoscine was less often realized, though the seeds of *Datura* in admixture with *Cannabis* were smoked for pleasure and for divinatory purposes, and this practice continues today in Indo-China and parts of Africa.

It was in the New World that *Datura* species were most used as sacred plants. There are numerous species in South America, including *D. suaveolens*, *D. aurea*, *D. candida*, *D. dolichocarpa*, *D. vulcanicola*, and *D. sanguinea*. All of these have been (and in most instances still are) used by the Indians. In Chapter 1 the use of *Datura* for infanticide and mass murders associated with royal burials was mentioned, and Hernandez mentioned the widespread use by the Aztecs of toaloatzin or tolohuaihuitl, which were based on extracts of various *Datura* species, for the treatment of rheumatism and for divination. He also warned that it caused madness.

The Mexican Indians still employ toloache, usually in combination with mescal, a strong liquor made from the *Agave*, but they use it as an intoxicant and hallucinogen rather than for magico-religious activities. These properties also endear the genus to the Indians of the American South-west, and the Navajo, Zuni, Paiute, Zunis, and others all have folklore associated with the visions induced by *Datura*. It is interesting to note that many of these include animals, and hallucinations involving animals are also a frequent manifestation of the witches' brews, suggesting that this is a 'trademark' of hyoscine intoxication.

Plants of the related genus *Brugmansia* are also widely used in the western parts of South America, and have a long association with man. These also contain tropane alkaloids, especially hyoscine, and the plant extracts seem to be particularly valued because they allow the users to commune with their ancestors. A nineteenth-century explorer gave the following description of the use of such an extract. 'In the course of a half of an hour, his eyes began to roll, foam issued from his mouth, and his whole body was agitated by frightful convulsions. After these violent symptoms had passed, a profound sleep of several hours duration followed, and when the subject had recovered, he related the particulars of his visit with his forefathers.'

The American cleric Cotton Mather, who was one of the first serious compilers of America folk medicine, gave a picturesque description of *Datura* intoxication in his book *The Christian Philosopher* (1720):

> *In Virginia there is a plant called the Jamestown weed [jimsonweed,* Datura stramonium*], whereof some having eaten plentifully became fools for several days, one would blow up a feather in the air, another sit naked, like a monkey, grinning at the rest, or fondly kiss and paw his companions, and sneer in their faces.*

Clearly these effects of lassitude and hallucinations are those that precede the narcosis induced by hyoscine.

A more recent description was provided by Carlos Castenada in 1968. He used *Datura* 'flying ointment' given to him by the Yaqui Indians of northern Mexico, and recorded his sensations:

> *The motion of my body was slow and shaky ... I looked down and saw don Juan sitting below me, way below me. The momentum carried me forward one more step, which was even more elastic and longer than the preceding one. And from there I soared ... I saw the dark sky above me, and the clouds going by me ... I enjoyed such freedom and swiftness as I had never known before.*

Finally, extracts of *Datura fastuosa* are used by many tribes in contemporary Africa for trials by ordeal and for complex puberty rites. In the latter, pubescent girls are dosed with the hallucinogen as part of ceremonies involving flagellation and ceremonial deflowering.

New World psychotropic plants and fungi

While *Datura* has found almost universal use, the trio of sacred preparations known to the Aztecs as ololiuqui, teonanacatl, and peyotl were (and are) used solely in the New World. There is evidence from ceramic relics that psychotropic plants and mushrooms have been used by the inhabitants of Mexico, Central America, and South America for at least three thousand years, but the first documentary evidence of their use was provided by Hernández and the Franciscan friar Bernardino de Sahagún. This chapter began with a quotation from Hernández's *Rerum Medicarum Novae Hispaniae Thesaurus*, but the classic *Historia general de las cosas de la Nueva España* of de Sahagún is in many ways an even more interesting work. In 1557 he began to investigate the Aztec culture, including the plants that they used for divination and other magico-religious purposes. All of his interviews had to be carried out in Nahuatl, the Aztec language, and his results were duly recorded (in Nahuatl) in what came to be called the *Florentine Codex*. This was the forerunner of the Spanish version referred to above, and it contains descriptions of ololiuqui, teonanacatl, peyotl, and several other magical brews.

The Inquisition also made 'valuable studies' in the new colonies, and from the reports of trials of Indians more information about the divinatory properties of local plant preparations were collected. But most of our information comes from the Mexican Instituto Medico Nacional at the turn of the century, and more recently from the writings of R. Gordon Wasson and Richard Evans Schultes. These two spent years with the Indians studying ethnobotany and ethnopharmacology locally, talking to shamans and watching them in action, and collecting and cataloguing the various psychotropic plant species. From these investigations several general features of aboriginal use can be identified.

Initially it was the lower castes who made the discoveries, presumably by accident, of psychotropic plants; but this knowledge was then absorbed by the shamans who concealed it from the rest of the tribe. This was achieved by imbuing the plants with divinity, and surrounding their use with elaborate and mysterious rituals. For example, even to this day, it is usual for a shaman and any recipient of a sacred brew to fast and abstain from sex before its consumption, and the actual consumption usually occurs at night or in darkness to the accompaniment of monotonous chanting by the shaman.

In addition, there is a strict hierarchy among shamans and their apprentices or assistants, and this was probably always the case. In present-day Mexico there are, in addition to shamans, *brujos* (witch-doctors), who also belong to the nobility of a community, and *yerberos* (herbalists) and *curanderos* (healers) who are from the peasant class. These peasant medicine men collect medicinal plants and actually treat patients, while the shamans and brujos are more concerned with magic and divination.

Finally, despite the introduction of Christianity four centuries ago, and the omnipotence of the Catholic church in Central and South America, the magico-religious practices of the Aztecs are still widespread. The major concession is that some of the sacred preparations now carry the names of saints, and much of the incantation invokes the names of the Virgin Mary, and Saint Peter and Saint Paul.

Ololiuqui

Ololiuqui was undoubtedly one of the most important Aztec magical brews, and its use in divinatory activities, in sacrificial ceremonies, and even as an aphrodisiac is well documented. It was prepared from the seeds of the morning glory plant *Rivea corymbosa*, and most accounts of its use speak of intoxication and hallucinations. This account from a sixteenth century Spanish missionary is typical: 'The natives communicate with the devil, for they usually talk when they become intoxicated with ololiuqui, and they are deceived by various hallucination which they attribute to the deity which they say resides in the seeds.'

Several other types of morning glory were probably used, but of these *Ipomoea violacea* (tlitliltzin to the Aztecs) was the most valued. Seeds of these two plants are still widely used in parts of Mexico, and are known in the Zapotec tongue as *badoh* (brown) from *Rivea corymbosa* and *badoh negro* (black) from *Ipomoea violacea*. Christian names are also used, such as *semilla de la Virgen* (seed of the Virgin) and *Hierba Maria*.

It was studies of this twentieth century use that enabled the ethnobotanists Wasson and Schultes to identify these plants as the source of ololiuqui and tlitliltzin. In the late 1950s, Wasson provided Albert Hofmann with some seeds from *Rivea corymbosa*, and to his amazement he found among their chemical constituents lysergic acid amides closely similar in structure to lysergic acid diethylamide (LSD), which he had synthesized in 1938. Hofmann had been engaged upon a general investigation of the ergot alkaloids derived from *Claviceps purpurea*, mentioned in Chapter 1. All of these were related in structure to lysergic acid (first synthesized by Jacobs and Craig in 1934), and some of them had proven clinical efficacy in obstetrics (see Chapter 3). Hofmann chose to prepare lysergic acid diethylamide (LSD) because it bore a structural similarity to coramine, a central nervous system stimulant. During these experiments in 1943 he experienced remarkable restlessness combined with a slight dizziness which forced him to abandon his work and go home. He described his subsequent experiences thus:

> *I sank into a not unpleasant intoxicated-like condition, characterized by an extremely stimulated imagination. In a dreamlike state ... I perceived an uninterrupted stream of fantastic pictures, extraordinary shapes with intense, kaleidoscopic play of colours.*

This experience induced him to consume 0.25 mg of LSD, which we now know to be a relatively large dose of this highly potent drug. This time the experience was more alarming:

Everything in my field of vision wavered and was distorted . . . Pieces of furniture assumed grotesque, threatening forms . . . The lady next door . . . was no longer Mrs R. but rather a malevolent, insidious witch with a coloured mask . . . A demon had invaded me, had taken possession of my body, mind, and soul. I jumped up and screamed, trying to free myself from him, but then sank down again and lay helpless on the sofa . . . I was seized by a dreadful fear of going insane.

Although the constituents of the *Rivea* species (lysergic acid amide and N-methyl-N-hydroxyethyl-lysergic acid amide) are about twenty times less potent than LSD, the origins of the hallucinogenic effects experienced by the Aztecs and their descendants was clearly revealed. The occurrence of ergot alkaloids outside of the fungal kingdom was of great chemotaxonomic interest, since it is usual for different plant and fungal species to produce widely differing chemical structures. Other researchers subsequently demonstrated that the various *Ipomoea* species also contained lysergic acid amides.

But the story does not end there. Hofmann and Wasson went on to speculate about the involvement of ergot alkaloids in magico-religious ceremonies in ancient Greece. In a book entitled *The Road to Eleusis*, written in collaboration with the Greek scholar Carl Ruck, they provided a most plausible explanation for the 4000 year old Eleusinian mysteries. These took place each autumn just outside Athens, and appear to have been some kind of dramatic reconstruction of the story of Persephone. One of the Greek myths tells how she was drugged and then abducted to the underworld by Hades, only to return in triumph with a son conceived while in that spiritual realm. Those who observed this drama had to participate in a lengthy initiation phase beforehand, and this included fasting and sexual abstinence, as well as the consumption of a wine spiked with what appears to have been barley just before the drama. Although the audience was sworn to secrecy, enough information about what ensued has been preserved to indicate that what they observed was awesome and visually very exciting. Wasson and Hofmann speculate that the barley was contaminated with ergot alkaloids of fungal origin, just as rye was infected in instances of ergotism. The Eleusinian mysteries were thus viewed by an audience who were suffering visual hallucinations. Certainly the parallels with the Aztec ceremonies are very striking: the secrecy, the abstinence, the consumption of a magical brew, and finally the mystical experience. We can never be certain if Wasson and Hofmann are right, but as a piece of ethnopharmacological detective work the book is fascinating and their evidence is persuasive.

As to the pharmacology of the lysergic acid amides, they appear to act at certain serotonin receptors on neurons in the mid-brain. In small amounts LSD is a serotonin mimic, but at larger doses it antagonizes the effects of the neurotransmitter. This is crucial, because these serotonin-dependent neurons connect with other noradrenalin-dependent neurons that are intimately involved in the regulation of behavioural responses to sensory stimulation. So it appears that the enormous changes in sensory perception associated with the use of LSD are due to disruption of the communication between these two sets of neurons. In particular, this may account for the fact that users experience a kind of 'scrambling of the senses' and may even feel that they have stepped outside of their own bodies.

In addition to visual and other sensory distortion, there is usually an increase in blood pressure, sweating, rapid breathing with palpitation of the heart, and very often significant changes in mood accompanied by great fear or manic excitement. In some users there are episodes which resemble the schizophrenic state, and there have been numerous fatalities associated with such 'bad trips'. During the 1960s, Timothy Leary, a lecturer in clinical psychology at Harvard University, did much to popularize the myth that consumption of LSD allowed consumers to examine their spirituality. He thus helped to found the hippy movement, which espoused love and peace and had a predilection for highly coloured (psychedelic) clothes and cars. The Beatles' song *Lucy in the Sky with Diamonds* with its 'tangerine trees and marmalade skies' was perhaps one of the most famous products of an LSD trip.

Leary was duly sacked by Harvard in 1963, and he proceeded to found the League for Spiritual Discovery in Mexico, where the use of LSD was viewed as a kind of sacrament akin to the Eucharist in Roman Catholic services. The manifesto for Leary's 'neurological politics' was quite explicit:

> *We, therefore, God-loving, life-loving, fun-loving men and women, appealing to the Supreme Judge of the Universe for the rectitude of our intentions, do ... solemnly publish and declare that we are free and independent, and that we are absolved from all Allegiance to the United States Government and all governments controlled by the menopausal.*

Not surprisingly, the US Government viewed the whole operation as subversive.

Despite its somewhat chequered past, LSD has been used therapeutically in psychiatric institutions, for the treatment of schizophrenics and those patients suffering from the effects of repressed traumatic experiences.

The lysergic acid amides are among the most potent hallucinogens known, and they exert their effects in doses of a few micrograms per kilogram of body weight. In contrast, the major psychoactive constituents of teonanacatl, psilocybin, and psilocin, produce similar effects at a dose of hundreds of micrograms per kilogram of body weight; and mescaline from the peyote cactus must be taken in quantities of tens of milligrams per kilogram. These psychedelics will be described in the following sections.

Teonanacatl

Just as there was a mushroom cult in the Old World, so there is good evidence that a similar cult existed in the New World. Numerous mushroom-shaped stones have been unearthed in Guatemala, and the most ancient of these is believed to be more than 3000 years old. With their hemispherical caps and intricately carved stems, these stones were originally thought to have been phallic symbols associated with a fertility cult. However, in the writing of de Sahagún there are several references to a mushroom god and to the use of a sacred mushroom known as *teonanacatl* (or God's flesh).

The Catholic Church was not slow to condemn the practice of communing with gods through the agency of magical preparations, and Cortes had the records concerning ololiuqui, teonanacatl, and peyotl destroyed. One missionary describing the use of teonanacatl stated that: 'When they are eaten, they intoxicate, depriving those who partake of them of their senses and making them believe a thousand absurdities.' And other authors related how the mushrooms caused hilarity and the induction of hallucinations.

Despite the wealth of archaeological artefacts and archival information, the identity of the fungal species was in doubt until the 1950s. Wasson and his wife made several trips to southern Mexico between 1953 and 1955 and studied the contemporary use of psychotropic fungi. However, only on a later trip in 1956 with a mycologist, Roger Heim, was an identification made. All of the sacred mushrooms were assigned to the genus *Psilocybe*, and *P. mexicana* was subsequently cultivated in the laboratories of the Museum National d'Histoire Naturelle in Paris. Once again Albert Hofmann was called in to assist with the pharmacological and chemical evaluations, and after several failures with animal models Hofmann agreed to a personal trial of the mushrooms. He consumed thirty-two dried specimens of *P. mexicana* weighing about 2.4 g, which was reckoned to be an average dose for the Mexican Indians. The records in his laboratory notebook provide a classic description of mushroom intoxication:

> *Thirty minutes after taking the mushrooms the exterior world began to undergo a strange transformation. Everything assumed a Mexican character ... Whether my eyes were closed or open I saw only Mexican motifs and colours. When the doctor supervising the experiment bent over me to check my blood pressure, he was transformed into an Aztec priest and I would not have been astonished if he had drawn an obsidian knife ... At the peak of the intoxication ... the rush of interior pictures, mostly abstract motifs rapidly changing in shape and colour, reached such an alarming degree that I feared that I would be torn into this whirlpool of form and colour and would dissolve. After about six hours the dream came to an end.*

Subsequent chemical investigations provided samples of the main psychotropic constituents, psilocybin and small amounts of psilocin, and both of these are close structural relatives of serotonin. Although psilocybin has only about 1 per cent of the potency of LSD, its subjective effects are very similar to those of LSD.

The mushroom cult is still very important in parts of Mexico, especially amongst the Mazatec Indians, and a complex ritual must be observed during the collection and consumption of the mushrooms. As usual the ceremony takes the form of a seance, and the shaman may chant for hours while beating his (or her) thighs rhythmically in time with his chanting. Schultes witnessed several such ceremonies, especially those supervised by the famous Mazatec shaman, Maria Sabina. In his book *Plants of the Gods* (with co-author Hofmann) he recorded her evocative description of teonanacatl intoxication:

> *The more you go inside the world of Teonanacatl, the more things are seen. And you also see our past and our future ... I knew and saw God: an immense clock that ticks, the spheres that go slowly around, and inside the stars, the earth, the entire universe, the day and the night, the cry and the smile, the happiness and the pain. .*

This description of what was clearly an unearthly experience helps to explain the survival of the cult during the last three thousand years.

Peyotl

It is likely that the peyote cactus has also been used as a source of hallucinogens for thousands of years. Dried samples have been found in ancient cliff dwellings in Texas, and various ceramic relics also support such antiquity. This spineless cactus, *Lophophora williamsii*, is widespread in Mexico, and it has a greenish-grey crown atop a parsnip-like root. The crown is sliced from the root and dried to form so-called 'mescal buttons', which can be kept more or less indefinitely without loss of psychoactive potency.

As so often, de Sahagún provided one of the first descriptions of peyote use:

> *There is another herb . . . of the earth. It is called peiotl. It is white. It is found in the north country. Those who eat or drink it see visions either frightful or laughable.*

As can be imagined, the Spanish were horrified to see enacted pagan practices in which something resembling the Eucharist of the Catholic mass was consumed; but despite countless attempts at suppression, the consumption of peyotl continued. Some attempts to marry the two cultures were made, including the establishment of a mission, El Santo de Jesus Peyotes, in the state of Coahuila in 1692. Here the wafers of peyotl and those of the Eucharist seem to have been used interchangeably, and this concession to a native religion was even more complete in the case of the Native American Church.

Some time around 1880 the peyote cult was imported into North America, most probably by Indians of the Kiowa and Comanche tribes returning from raiding parties in Mexico. During the next forty years, the cult spread throughout the South-western States and among the tribes of the Great Plains. Various modes of worship evolved, in part Christian and in part pagan, and numerous attempts were made by the US authorities to have peyote banned, without success. Several bizarre court cases were conducted, but failed to prove that the drug was associated with drunken behaviour or licentiousness. Most Indian defendants claimed that they took peyote in order to commune with God, and through his help become better persons. In particular, there was very good evidence that the consumption of peyote helped these reservation Indians to become abstemious from alcohol.

Such encouragement to sobriety was hardly the mark of a dangerous narcotic drug, and although persecution persisted the growing numbers of adherents of the Native American Church continued to use peyote. In 1962 the American Civil Liberties Union won a test case against the State of California, which was contesting the religious importance of peyote. Finally in 1967 the US Congress voted to protect the religious liberty of the quarter of a million adherents, and legalized the use of peyote as a sacrament. As a result mescal buttons can be obtained quite legally via mail order and are widely used for medico-religious purposes by North American Indians.

The cactus contains at least fifteen alkaloids of varying psychoactivity, but the most important of these is mescaline. It was first isolated in pure form in 1896, but the first pseudo-scientific investigations were carried out on the crude peyote slices. Thus, in the same year American neurologist Weir Mitchell described the 'brilliant visions' induced by consumption of the drug. A more detailed description of peyote intoxication was provided by the British psychologist Havelock Ellis.

He made a concoction of three peyote buttons and water, and drank this over a period of two hours. At first he felt a little nauseous and light-headed, but then the hallucinations began. In his account for the *Contemporary Review* of January 1898, he recalled:

> *Visions became distinct but still indescribable—mostly a vast field of golden jewels, studded with red and green stones, ever changing. This moment was, perhaps, the most delightful of the experience, for at the same time the air around me seemed flushed with vague perfumes, producing with the visions a delicious effect ... a kind of removal from earthly cares and the appearance of a purely internal life which excites astonishment.*

Subsequent experiments were carried out with pure mescaline, and probably the most extensive study took place at the Maudsley Hospital, London, in 1930. Dr Eric Guttman supplied mescaline to sixty healthy volunteers and then collated their experiences. Most of them described the usual distortions of time and space, and brilliant visual hallucinations, but one of the most entertaining accounts was of an object 'like an iridescent plum pudding suspended in the sky exactly a hundred miles above the earth' which then turned into an Aztec figure.

Aldous Huxley also tried mescaline (about 0.4 g) as part of his wider interests in spiritualism and religion. In his book *The Doors of Perception* he gave a literary account of what he described as 'the miracle, moment by moment, of naked existence' and a 'sacramental vision of reality'. He experienced all of the usual phenomena, but for him it was the altered perceptions of everyday objects that were most remarkable. He observed furniture and pictures as if he was actually part of them. Of a chair with bamboo legs he says: 'How miraculous their tubularity, how supernatural their polished smoothness!' A famous self-portrait of Cézanne became a 'small goblin-like man looking out through a window in the page before me.' But perhaps most astutely he observed that mescaline allows the user to 'experience only the heavenly side of schizophrenia', unlike the much more potent LSD, which he tried on his deathbed.

The spectrum of pharmacological activity of mescaline is broadly similar to that of LSD, though it has only about 0.2 per cent of the hallucinogenic potency. However, despite its similarity in structure to the catecholamines, mescaline has very little effect on their receptors. Its very simple structure has attracted the illicit chemists, and both synthetic mescaline and related 'designer drug' structures have been prepared by back-street operators. Of the latter designer drugs, DOM (or 2,5-dimethoxy-4-methylamphetamine), with a potency about 100-fold greater than mescaline, was the most popular during the hippy era of the 1960s. More recently (in the 1980s), MMDA or Ecstasy (3-methoxy-4,5-methylenedioxyamphetamine) has become very popular. Recent research with rats has shown that Ecstasy is neurotoxic and destroys nerve-endings. Although these nerve-endings regenerate following removal of the drug, they are anatomically different from unaffected neurons. Long-term use of Ecstasy is thus fraught with danger.

But this pseudo-sophisticated use of mescaline and analogues should be considered alongside the complex rituals of collection and consumption of peyote that are still practised by the Huichol Indians of Mexico. These are eloquently described by Hofmann and Schultes in their book *Plants of the Gods*. Once a year the shaman leads pilgrims on a peyote hunt, and all abstain from sex, food, and sleep for the duration of the journey. The collected peyote is consumed at various festivals throughout the year, but most importantly at the time of the annual planting. Celebrants may dance and chant for several days under the influence of peyote, and supplication is made to the gods to ensure healthy crops and a bountiful harvest.

The peyote services held by the Kiowa and Comanche are less exotic but probably more frequent. They are held at Christmas, Thanksgiving, Easter, etc., as well as to celebrate the birth of a child or a safe return. These are deeply felt religious experiences, and as J. S. Slotkin (who wrote a book entitled the *Peyote Religion*, based upon his time on the Menomini Indian reservation) so aptly put it: 'The white man goes into his church house and talks about Jesus; the Indian goes into his teepee and talks to Jesus.'

Mescaline is also the major psychoactive substance present in the tall, columnar cactus *Trichocereus pachanoi* to the extent of about 1.3 g per kilogram of fresh plant material. This has been an important magical plant in Peru since at least 100 BC, though archaeological evidence indicates that it may have been in use as early as 1300 BC. Much of the renowned artwork of the Mochican civilization, which flourished between 100 BC and AD 700, is believed to depict shamanistic activities involving this cactus. It is still widely used throughout Peru and Bolivia and is usually known as San Pedro. The cactus is sliced and then boiled in water, usually in admixture with *Datura arborea*, to produce a drink that is valued for its medicinal and magical properties.

Ayahuasca (caapi)

Amongst the Indians of the north-western parts of South America—those areas of Brazil, Colombia, and Ecuador that lie between the Amazon and the Orinoco rivers—*ayahuasca* (or 'vine of the soul') is the most important magical brew. Its potency as an aid to prophecy and divination is legendary, to the extent that when its major constituent was first isolated it was christened 'telepathine'.

It is obtained from vines of the *Banisteriopsis* genus, especially the species *B. caapi* and *B. inebrans*, and the bark is either boiled with water or pulverized in cold water to produce an intoxicating liquid. The first reports of its use were given in the 1850s by the English botanist Richard Spruce, who spent the period between 1849 and 1864 exploring the Amazon region and the Andes. He sent numerous samples of plants back to Kew Gardens for identification and cataloguing, and his description of the effects of ayahuasca suggest a more frightening experience than those produced by peyotl or teonanacatl. He reported that, soon after consuming the brew, the Indians saw 'beautiful lakes, woods laden with fruit, birds of brilliant plumage', but then 'the Indian turns deadly pale, trembles in every limb, and horror is in his aspect', then shortly afterwards 'he bursts into a perspiration, and seems possessed with reckless fury, seizes whatever arms are at hand . . . and rushes to the doorway, where he inflicts violent blows on the ground or the doorposts, calling out all the while, "Thus would I do to mine enemy X were this he!" In about ten minutes the excitement has passed off, and the Indian grows calm, but appears exhausted.'

He does not record his own experience of ayahuasca, possibly because

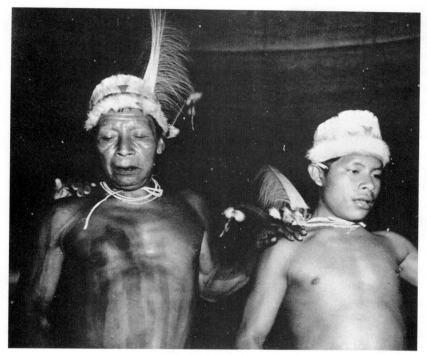

A shaman and his pupil intoxicated with ayahuasca (caapi). The brew obtained from vines of the *Banisteriopsis* genus is commonly used by Indians of the north-west Amazonian region. (From the personal collection of Richard Evans Schultes, Emeritus Director, the Botanical Museum, Harvard University.)

he was forced to consume a local beer and palm wine at the same time, and also forced to smoke a cigar 'two feet long and thick as a wrist'. This left him with a 'strong inclination to vomit'. Others have reported intensely coloured visions, especially of jaguars and large snakes; and the Indians claim that their night vision is greatly improved, thus allowing them to run through the forest at night without endangering themselves.

The psychotropic alkaloids present in the brew include harmine and harmaline, and these have at least a partial structural resemblance to serotonin. Their pharmacological effect is thus likely to be due to blockade of serotonin receptors in the brain, and they are certainly cross-reactive with LSD and psilocybin, which also have this activity. In addition they inhibit the oxidative metabolism of other brain amines, so causing a more generalized disturbance of central nervous system function, and this explains why some forms of ayahuasca are more potent than others. Frequently the brews are deliberately contaminated with *Banisteriopsis rusbyana* or the aptly named *Psychotria viridis*, and these contain the hallucinogen N,N-dimethyltryptamine, again a structural relative of serotonin. This cocktail of psychoactive substances ensures that the effects of ayahuasca intoxication are prolonged and intensified, but in addition the recipient may become reckless or even aggressive.

A particularly graphic description of ayahuasca intoxication was provided by Franklin Flores, professor of botany at the University in Iquitos, Peru. He drank the brew on at least thirty occasions during the period 1972–4 as part of ethnopharmacological studies on the local Indian brews. He reported: 'Suddenly the panorama of darkness becomes a vast moving spiral. One is thrust, crying, into this spiral, a terrifying experience.' This first phase of hallucinations lasted about ten minutes, and was followed by visions of grotesque human and animal forms: 'A female patient visualized a large boa (constrictor) coming towards her . . . She was powerless to move, while the boa coiled around her body. Her screams were terrifying . . . Eventually the animal retreated and she became calm.' Hearing became very acute: '. . . the voice of a female friend who recently died suddenly and clearly was heard, soft at first but soon building into a high-pitched crescendo that seemingly never stopped.'

Finally, both harmine and harmaline cause sexual excitation in laboratory rats, and the aphrodisiac potential of ayahuasca should not be dismissed. Certainly, it is widely used in initiation rites for adolescent boys, and these ceremonies often involve flagellation and other more overtly sexual activities.

Hallucinogenic snuffs

In some parts of South America vines of the *Banisteriopsis* genus are used in the form of a snuff, but it is the hallucinogenic snuffs from around sixty species of *Virola* and yopo from *Anadenanthera peregrina* that are of most ethnopharmacological interest.

Once again we have Richard Spruce to thank for most of the early information about yopo or niopo, though a missionary in Colombia wrote in 1560: 'The Indians are accustomed to take Yopo and Tobacco . . . they become drowsy while the devil, in their dreams, shows them all the vanities and corruptions he wishes them to see.' Both Spruce and the explorer Baron von Humboldt described how the snuff was prepared from the seeds of the legume *Anadenanthera peregrina*, and Spruce went so far as to purchase the equipment (a kind of pestle and mortar) needed to grind the seeds. He also bought the rest of the paraphernalia:

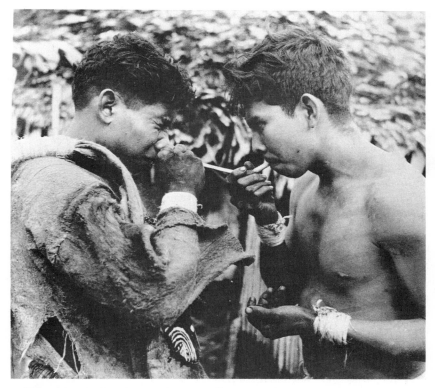

Colombian Indian boys taking snuff. (From the personal collection of Richard Evans Schultes, Emeritus Director, the Botanical Museum, Harvard University.)

The snuff is kept in a mull made of a bit of the leg-bone of the jaguar ... For taking the snuff, they use an apparatus made of the leg bones of herons or other long-shanked birds put together in the shape of the letter Y. *The lower tube being inserted in the snuff-box and the knobs in the nostrils, the snuff is forcibly inhaled, with the effect of narcotizing a novice, or indeed a practised hand if taken in sufficient quantity.*

The apparatus was duly sent to Kew Gardens where it still resides in the museum.

The snuff produces an immediate effect. The muscles of the face twitch, and the recipient may then behave in an aggressive way before suffering a loss of coordination, followed by stupor, during which nightmarish hallucinations are experienced. Or as one nineteenth century observer wrote: 'His eyes started from his head, his mouth contracted, his limbs trembled . . . He was obliged to sit down or he would have fallen. He was drunk, but only for about five minutes; he was then gayer.'

The Waika people, who inhabit the north-western parts of Brazil and neighbouring areas of Colombia and Venezuela, take frequent overdoses of this snuff, and also make much use of *Virola* snuffs. Schultes spent time with these Indians in the mid-1960s, and reported that as much as three to six teaspoons of snuff was consumed per inhalation. The effects are similar to those produced by yopo, with hyperexcitability followed by stupor, and the Indians believe that they see the 'little people' in their nightmarish dreams.

Schultes provided very detailed observations on the preparation of *Virola* snuffs, and it is clear that the psychoactive substances are present in the bark. The Indians carefully strip the bark from the tree and collect the red exudate, which is then usually boiled (to destroy metabolic enzymes) before concentration. The resultant dry red mass is pulverized to yield the snuff. Many species of *Virola* are used but *V. theidora* is pre-eminent. All of these snuffs contain various dimethyltryptamines (structural relatives of serotonin) as their major psychoactive components. The most active of these has about 0.1 per cent of the hallucinogenic potency of LSD.

Tobacco

The explorer Richard Spruce also recorded native use of tobacco in conjunction with the various snuffs described in the last section. He wrote:

When the payé [medicine man] is called in to treat a patient, he first snuffs up his nose such a quantity of niopo as suffices to throw him into a sort of ecstasy, wherein he professes to divine the nature of the evil wish which has caused the sickness, and to gather force to counteract it. He next lights a very thick cigar of tobacco, inhales a quantity of smoke, and puffs it out over the sick man . . . This done, the payé professes to suck out the ill, by applying his mouth to the seat of the pain . . . and he spits out the morbid matter—most likely tobacco or coca juice—and sometimes produces from his mouth thorns and other substances . . . which he pretends to have extracted from the sick man's body.

Four centuries earlier one can imagine the incredulity of Columbus's men when they first observed Indians in Cuba inserting smouldering leaves of *Nicotiana tabacum* into their mouths and nostrils. Sir Walter Raleigh was likewise fascinated when he arrived in Virginia. The plant variety native to Virginia was *N. rustica* and this was inferior in terms of the tobacco produced to the South American variety *N. tabacum*. It was this latter variety that was subsequently cultivated by the European settlers in Virginia.

Within 150 years tobacco smoking was well established throughout Western Europe, and as usual much of the early success of this new product was due to its supposed aphrodisiac properties. Opposition to the new habit varied from country to country. In China, Japan, and Persia smoking was prohibited and those caught smoking were executed. James I of England, who had Sir Walter Raleigh executed (though not solely for his introduction of tobacco), wrote a pamphlet entitled *A Counterblast to Tobacco*. In this he described smoking as 'a custom loathsome to the Eye, hateful to the Nose, harmful to the Braine, dangerous to the Lungs, and in the black stinking fumes thereof, nearest resembling the horrible Stygian Smoke of the Pit that is bottomless'.

The major active constituent of tobacco is nicotine, named after Jean Nicot who helped to popularize the use of tobacco smoke in the sixteenth century as a treatment for headache. Nicotine was first isolated in pure form in 1828, but its pharmacological effects were not demonstrated until 1898. The Cambridge physiologist Langley painted nicotine solution on to the autonomic ganglia from various animal species and observed an initial stimulation followed by inhibition of nerve transmission. He was, in fact, the first to propose the idea of the autonomic nervous system with its sympathetic and parasympathetic components, and his research led ultimately to the recognition of the discrete nicotinic subclass of acetylcholine receptors. Each cigarette puff contains up to 350 micrograms of nicotine, and the pleasurable effects of smoking are due to the interaction of the drug with nicotinic receptors in the brain. Not surprisingly classic withdrawal symptoms are experienced by habitual smokers when they attempt to stop smoking. Despite the obvious dangers of tobacco smoking, so vigorously described by James I, this ancient South American custom shows no sign of dying out. Although smoking is now less popular in the developed world, the habit is growing in popularity in the developing countries, owing primarily to aggressive advertising and marketing.

Nutmeg

Before the advent of refrigeration spoilage of food was a perennial problem, and it is usually assumed that one incentive for the early voyages of discovery was the quest for spices that would obscure the flavour of putrified food. It was subsequently discovered that many of these food additives had gastrointestinal carminative properties, or would keep intestinal worms at bay. In addition it has been suggested that the psychotropic potential of some of these spices was also a reason for their popularity. But whatever the motives for the rapid rise of the spice trade, there is no doubting the importance and the lucrative nature of the trade.

The maritime state of Venice was pre-eminent in the field from the ninth century to the fall of Constantinople in 1453. For the next century Portugal dominated the trade in the East, while the Spaniards sent Columbus to find a new westerly route to the rich spice islands of the East. It was the Portuguese who discovered the Banda Islands off Indonesia in 1512, and the tree *Myristica fragrans* which was native to the islands. The apricot-like fruit of this tree contains a brown seed—the nutmeg—and it is the volatile oil from the seed that imparts the heavy aroma characteristic of this spice.

Though the Portuguese made the initial discovery, it was the Dutch who made the importation of nutmegs into a massive commercial enterprise. They dominated the East Indian trade during the seventeenth century, and for a while Amsterdam was the only port from which nutmeg could be obtained. It is easy to comprehend the great popularity of this spice, since it was imbued with aphrodisiac, soporific, or abortifacient properties, depending upon which authority one believes.

The botanist Löbel provided the first written report (in 1576) of its inebriating properties, and he claimed that 'a pregnant English lady who, having eaten ten or twelve nutmegs, became deliriously inebriated'. Johannes Purkinje, famous for his numerous discoveries in cellular biology, ate three nutmegs in 1829, and claimed that the resultant intoxication was similar to that which he had already experienced with *Cannabis*. In the 1970s, prisoners in US jails experimented with powdered nutmeg and hot milk concoctions, though the 'trip' was usually not good enough to justify the suffering caused by the subsequent hangover.

Nutmeg contains no known psychoactive compounds, and its intoxicating properties cannot yet be explained. The volatile oil contains two major constituents, elemecin and myristicin, in a ratio of about 1:3, and it has been suggested that these might be converted after ingestion into molecules that are structural relatives of the amphetamines. This would require the addition of ammonia, and although it is feasible this transformation has never been observed.

At this point it is worth mentioning something about the amphetamines. The original member of this family of synthetic drugs (amphetamine) was first prepared in 1897, but the discovery in 1928 of its ability to cause a prolonged increase in blood pressure, led to its introduction as a stimulant. During World War II it was widely used (as benzedrine) together with the more active methylamphetamine (methedrine) to alleviate the symptoms of battle fatigue. After the war the drugs became freely available in many parts of the world, and in the USA the use of methedrine ('speed', 'purple hearts') reached epidemic proportions in the late sixties. Drug addicts resorted to injection of crushed tablets and a large number of cases of paranoid schizophrenia resulted.

The mode of action of the amphetamines is similar to that of cocaine. They both inhibit re-uptake of neurotransmitters, and thus increase the amount of free noradrenalin in the brain and also peripherally. In controlled clinical doses they have a variety of useful effects, including increased alertness and mental clarity, reduction in fatigue, suppression of appetite (hence their use in slimming), and vasoconstriction, especially in engorged mucous membranes (hence their use as nasal decongestants).

Iboga

The West African plant *Tabernanthe iboga* provides an extract that has been described as the 'cocaine of Africa'. Certainly natives chew the roots of this plant to obtain relief from hunger and fatigue, but in larger amounts the extracted ibogaine is said to produce visual hallucinations and apparent levitation. As much as 300–800 g of dried bark may be chewed by shamans and other members of the tribe during religious festivals, and as one observer noted: 'The men began dancing around each of the poles in the temple—they jumped, stamped, leaped in a compulsive sort of way . . . [as the women] shook their rattles and sang.' As usual this intoxication is believed to be an adjunct to soothsaying and divination, but iboga is also claimed to have aphrodisiac properties.

In its pharmacological activity, ibogaine resembles the so-called tricyclic antidepressants like amitriptyline, and although there is some confusion over their mode of action it is probable that they produce a generalized disruption in re-uptake of the neurotransmitters noradrenalin and serotonin into neurons. This increases the availability of serotonin and noradrenalin in the central nervous system.

As for the reputed aphrodisiac activity of iboga, this is probably due to the alkaloid yohimbine which is present in *Alchornea floribunda*, a common adulterant of the iboga extracts. This probably acts by increasing the bood supply to the erectile tissues of the genitalia and also provides a central enhancement of the reflexes involved in the control of ejaculation.

Inebriants

Alcohol

A large number of plants provide extracts that have a psychotropic effect that falls short of hallucinogenic. They are usually described as intoxicating and their constituents are intoxicants or inebriants. The most important of these is alcohol (ethyl alcohol, or ethanol) from the fermentation of many kinds of fruits and cereals. Most wines are produced by fermentation of grapes from the various *Vitis* species, most notably *Vitis vinifera*.

There are numerous imaginative legends concerning the origins of viticulture (grape production) and oenology (wine production); but it is generally agreed that winemaking was first practised in the Middle East about 6000–8000 years ago. Wild vines still exist, like *Vitis silvestris* in Europe and *Vitis labrusca* in North America, and the modern wine-producing vines have been bred from these.

Wine consumption was already well established in ancient Egypt, and one of their most important gods, Osiris, was not only Lord of the Dead but also presided over viticulture. Dignitaries were buried with enough wine to sustain them on their journey to the after-world, and the mourners partook of the same liquid refreshment. The ancient Greeks were somewhat slow to adopt the techniques of oenology, and the many wild vines were mostly valued for the fruit they bore. Wine was imported from other countries, and often used solely for medicinal purposes, though eventually wine production became widely established in Attica and Thessaly. But it was the Romans who developed the art of winemaking, with the benefit of techniques and vines from all parts of their empire. At its zenith, Rome accounted for the consumption of around 25 million gallons of wine each year.

Britain had no native vines, or at least none was seen by Julius Caesar when he invaded Britain in 55 BC, although wine was being imported by the Belgae who inhabited the southern parts of Britain. After the Roman conquest vines were imported, and there is abundant archaeological evidence of Roman vineyards in many parts of Britain. By the time the Romans retreated from Gaul (*c.* fifth century AD) in response to the barbarian invasions of Italy, vineyards had been established near Paris, in Champagne and Languedoc, and alongside the rivers Moselle and Rhine.

In addition to these wines made wholly from grapes, the Moors prepared date wines, the Japanese made rice wines, the Indians of Mexico made *pulque* from the agave, the Vikings fermented honey to make mead, and the Incas made *chicha* from maize. This latter beverage was and is more like a beer than a wine, and its crudity owes something to its preparation. This involves women of the village masticating the kernels of corn, then spitting them into a communal pot where fermentation is allowed to proceed. The enzymes present in saliva help to break down the starch of the kernels, providing glucose for the airborne yeasts which effect the actual fermentation.

Modern beer brewing uses the yeast *Saccharomyces cerevisiae*, and wild yeasts were probably used by the Babylonians for making beer as long ago as 5000–6000 BC. The addition of hops (*Humulus lupulus*) and other bitter herbs is a much more recent invention, and they were initially added as preservatives rather than as flavourings. Beer drinking and drunkenness were a feature of ancient Egyptian life, and there are enough tomb paintings to establish that the brewing process was not dissimilar to that used today.

The Greeks learned their brewing skills from the Egyptians, and although the Romans were not great beer drinkers beer was the staple beverage of the tribes in the western part of their empire. Dioscorides noted that the Britons and the Hiberni (Irish) drank *courni* made from fermented barley; and Pliny was impressed that they had 'invented a method of making water itself intoxicate'.

Alehouses or *tabernae* were introduced during Saxon times, and were to be found at important resting places on the Roman roads in Britain. The Normans reintroduced the art of winemaking after the invasion of 1066, and thirty-eight vineyards are listed in the 'Domesday Book'. But beer drinking has always remained an important social pastime of the British. It is amusing to compare William of Malmesbury's comments (in the twelfth century) on social drinking with those that might be made about twentieth century party-goers: 'Drinking in particular, was a universal practice, in which occupation they passed entire nights as well as days . . . They were accustomed to eat till they became surfeited, and to drink till they were sick.'

As to the pharmacology of alcohol, it is one of the few psychotropic substances that most people have encountered. Mild intoxication occurs once a blood concentration of around 30–50 mg of alcohol per 100 ml of blood has been attained, and a state of mild euphoria is experienced. In those unaccustomed to alcohol, garrulity and uncharacteristic silly behaviour are often observed. Once the concentration has reached 100 mg per 100 ml, most individuals suffer more serious neurological disturbances, which result in slurred speech and a staggering gait. Silliness and even aggressive behaviour are also more likely, even in hardened drinkers.

Finally, at a concentration of 200 mg per 100 ml vision and movement are impaired; coma results at twice that concentration. Deaths from alcohol overdose are usually due to respiratory distress that accompanies the comatose state.

The actual mode of action of alcohol is not clear. It has an anaesthetic effect, so some degree of alteration of neurotransmission is obvious. However, it is acetaldehyde (ethanal), the main metabolite of ethanol, that is the likely cause of most of the problems. Acetaldehyde probably reacts with dopamine to produce salsolinol and with tryptamine to produce tetrahydroharman, both of which have psychotropic activity. Dopamine is the immediate precursor of noradrenalin, and was shown in 1958 to be a brain neurotransmitter in its own right, with a special involvement in those areas of the brain concerned with control of motor behaviour. A more detailed account of the pharmacology of dopamine will be given in Chapter 3.

Finally, the aphrodisiac or libido-enhancing effects of alcohol are often cited. Ogden Nash extolled the virtues of alcohol as an 'ice-breaker': 'Candy is dandy, but liquor is quicker'. And the much quoted comments of the porter in *Macbeth* (II, iii) are as apposite today as they were 300 years ago:

> *Lechery, sir, it provokes, and unprovokes; it provokes the desire, but it takes away the performance. Therefore much drink may be said to be an equivocator with lechery; it makes him, and it mars him; it sets him on, and it takes him off; it persuades him, and disheartens him; makes him stand to, and not stand to; in conclusion, equivocates him in a sleep, and, giving him the lie, leaves him.*

Kava

Although beer has largely replaced kava as the major intoxicating brew of Polynesia, kava bars are still quite common. This beverage made from the shrub *Piper methysticum* was for centuries venerated among the communities of the idyllic islands of Polynesia. It was originally prepared exclusively by children, who would collect the roots and lower stems of the shrub, chew them, and then spit the soggy mass into a communal bowl. The salivary enzymes were clearly important for release of the psychotropic constituents marindin and dihydromethysticin, from the vegetable matrix. The dried residue was then mixed with water and the extract was strained to produce kava. The mode of preparation is essentially the same today.

A measure equivalent to a half-full split coconut shell is sufficient to produce a state of well-being and somnolence, although larger quantities may induce a quarrelsome state and even drunken behaviour. This was too much for the missionaries, and they tried, with some success, to rid the islands of this unholy brew.

The mode of action of kava is completely unknown, though the chemical structures of the main constituents have some structural similarity to those from nutmeg, and like these they may be metabolized to amphetamine-like compounds.

Absinthe

Since the wine yeast cannot survive in solutions containing more than about 12–13 per cent of alcohol (ethyl alcohol, or ethanol), fortified wines and spirits were not available before the invention of distillation by the Arabs in the tenth century. The technique takes advantage of the fact that alcohol has a lower boiling point than water (78 °C versus 100 °C), and can thus be boiled out of an aqueous solution and condensed in a cooled receiver. Using this method it is impossible to obtain pure alcohol, because some water always co-distils with it, but solutions that contain up to about 95 per cent of ethanol by volume are attainable.

The manufacture of spirits like rum or whisky involves fermentation of a grain (sugar-cane and barley respectively), then distillation of the resultant wine-strength brew, such that the volatile flavours are concentrated in the alcohol. Liqueurs, by contrast, are usually produced by steeping fruits and/or herbs in brandy or vodka or a similar spirit, with subsequent filtration to remove the vegetable residues. Of all the innumerable spirits and liqueurs that man has devised, the pale-green liqueur absinthe is of incomparable interest.

The absinthe of the nineteenth century was made by steeping wormwood (*Artemesia absinthium, A. maritima,* or *A. pontica*), anise (*Pimpinella anisum*), and fennel (*Foeniculum vulgare*), together with lesser amounts of nutmeg, juniper, hyssop, etc., in 85 per cent alcohol, and then, after the addition of some water, distilling the resultant green brew. Additional herbs were often added to the distillate, and after filtration the highly alcoholic mixture was diluted with water to produce a liqueur with an alcohol content of about 75 per cent by volume.

Wormwood was certainly the most important ingredient from a psychotropic standpoint, since the thujone that it contains is apparently neuroactive, and certainly neurotoxic. The Ebers papyrus (*c.* 1500 BC) mentions wormwood, as did Hippocrates, Dioscorides, and Gerard ('wormewood voideth away the wormes of the guts'); and it seems to have

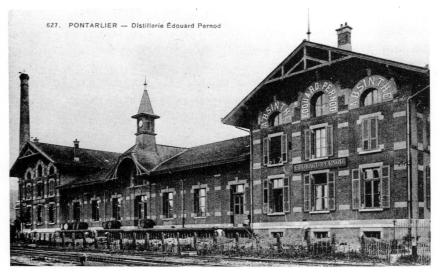

627. PONTARLIER — Distillerie Édouard Pernod

The Pernod distillery at Pontarlier was established in 1797 to manufacture absinthe, which was to become the social beverage of the nineteenth century. The aperitif *Pernod* produced today is based on the original recipe, but no longer contains any wormwood. (Photo: Late nineteenth century, reproduced by kind permission of J. Guiraud, Conservateur du Musée de Pontarlier, France.)

had general medicinal utility. Most ancient treatises record its value in the treatment of intestinal worms (hence the name), though various concoctions were used to treat rheumatism, anaemia, gout, jaundice, and as a 'comfort for hart and braine'. One of the earliest professional medicinal preparations was prescribed by Dr John Hill for his patients with gout. He produced tincture of wormwood by steeping flowers of the plant in brandy for six weeks.

But these teas and infusions were weak in comparison with absinthe itself, which is believed to have been invented in 1792 by a French doctor, Pierre Ordinaire, who lived as an exile in Switzerland. He was primarily interested in the medicinal properties of absinthe, but when he died the recipe passed into the hands of his landlady, who promptly opened a small absinthe shop. This excited the interest of a certain Major Henri Dubied, who was already taking absinthe as a remedy for indigestion and had noticed that it also enhanced his sexual performance. His son-in-law, Henri-Louis Pernod, had made the same discovery, and having purchased the recipe from Ordinaire's housekeeper they went into production in 1797.

Its popularity grew slowly, but it received a massive boost when the French army chose to use absinthe (and simpler wormwood extracts) to ward off disease during the North African campaigns of the 1840s. On their return to France, the soldiers retained the absinthe habit, and absinthe became established as the social beverage of the nineteenth century. When diluted with water, usually with the addition of a little sugar, a cloudy, pale-green mixture was produced with a bitter, aniseed flavour.

It was the drink of artists, writers, actors, and sculptors, including de Maupassant, Toulouse Lautrec, Dégas, Gauguin, van Gogh, Manet, Baudelaire, and Verlaine. Verlaine wrote that 'pour moi, ma gloire n'est qu'une absinthe humble éphèmere'. Oscar Wilde was more explicit:

> *After the first glass (of absinthe) you see things as you wish they were. After the second, you see things as they are not. Finally you see things as they really are, and that is the most horrible thing in the world.*

Many paintings of the period show absinthe drinkers, mostly depicted with a glazed expression, and writers spoke of the wild sensations (including those of sexual excitement) that absinthe elicited. In small amounts it was said to stimulate the mind and the sexual appetite, but in excessive amounts it produced terrifying hallucinations and eventually a condition termed 'absinthism'. Inveterate absinthists were pallid, enfeebled creatures, usually with signs and symptoms of mental derangement, and most of the aforementioned cultural figures died young or, like van Gogh, committed suicide.

The hazards of absinthe did not go unnoticed, and as early as the mid-1860s experiments with animals had shown that the liqueur induced convulsions and impaired respiration in dogs. But despite the publication of these and other results, the appetite for absinthe among the French increased dramatically towards the end of the nineteenth century, especially since a glass of absinthe cost less than a loaf of bread. By 1913 the French were consuming over ten million gallons of absinthe per year, and the amount of crime perpetrated by absinthists had reached alarming proportions.

The example of Jean Lanfray is not untypical. He was a notorious French alcoholic living in Switzerland and in the habit of drinking several absinthes per day, not to mention several bottles of his own home-made wine and some brandy. On 28 August 1905, at the end of his drinking day, he argued with his wife, then shot and killed her and his two daughters. In the subsequent trial his 'mental derangement' was ascribed to absinthism,

An advertisement for absinthe supposedly free of thujone, the neurotoxic constituent of wormwood. (Photo: Late nineteenth century, reproduced by kind permission of J. Guiraud, Conservateur du Musée de Pontarlier, France.)

and shortly afterwards the liqueur was banned in Switzerland. France finally banned absinthe in 1915, but the recipe survives in the form of the aperitifs Pernod and Ricard, though neither of these contains any wormwood. Absinthe is still made (illegally) near Neuchatel in Switzerland, and in Spain, which never banned the liqueur.

As to the mode of action of thujone very little is known. It is a stimulant of the autonomic nervous system, and in large doses it induces convulsions followed by loss of consciousness; but its long-term effects on the central nervous system and its role in the aetiology of absinthism are open to speculation. Many of the symptoms of absinthism also resemble those of alcoholism, and most absinthists were certainly alcoholics.

Perhaps the best poetic descriptions of absinthe (the 'Green Fairy') was provided by the French poet Arthur Rimbaud:

Je suis la Fée Verte,
Ma robe est couleur d'esperance...
Je suis la ruine et la douleur,
Je suis la honte,
Je suis le deshonneur,
Je suis la mort,
Je suis l'Absinthe.

However, in common with all of the other preparations described in this chapter, absinthe is derived from a plant that has a long association with folk medicine, and this topic is the subject of the final chapter of this book.

Medicine

Introduction: a history of pharmacy

> *O! mickle is the powerful grace that lies*
> *In herbs, plants, stones, and their true qualities:*
> *For nought so vile that on earth doth live*
> *But to the earth some special good doth give,*
> *Within the infant rind of this weak flower*
> *Poison hath residence and medicine power:*
>   Romeo and Juliet, II, iii

The ancients had discovered the dose-related effects of plants long before
Shakespeare wrote these much-quoted lines. For an example of this, one
has only to recall that the mandrake was used (according to dose) for
murder, magic, or medicine long before the time of Christ. The earliest
systematic study of herbal medicine was made by the Emperor Shên Nung,
a shadowy figure who probably lived about 3000 BC. His *Pen Tsao* ('Great
Herbal') mentioned the medicinal uses of 365 drugs. Of these, 120 were
non-toxic, 120 were mildly toxic, and 125 were unsuitable for prolonged
use. The plants included *Ephedra* species for bronchial problems, the
purgative *Ricinus communis*, and the opium poppy, *Papaver somniferum*.
These plants provide the clinically useful ephedrine (an early treatment for
asthma), castor oil, and morphine respectively.

The Assyrians left a legacy of 1500 years of herbal medicine (*c.* 1900 to

400 BC) in the form of 660 clay tablets that extolled the virtues of around 1000 medicinal plants; but it is the Ebers papyrus that provides the best insight into ancient pharmacy. This was written about 1500 BC, but only came to light in 1862 when the archaeologist Georg Ebers bought it from a wealthy Egyptian. This character claimed that the 1 by 68 ft scroll had been found between the knees of a mummy in one of the tombs at Thebes. Whatever its source, it was in perfect condition and provided a wealth of information about ancient Egyptian pharmacy and surgical practices. Over 800 remedies are described in it, involving the use of plant extracts, animal organs, and minerals, as well as much magic. These range from efficacious remedies 'to get rid of the excrement in the body of a person' (castor oil and beer) to obviously useless ones like 'an old book cooked in oil, smear on his body' (to rid a child of excess urine). If these formulations failed, there were a number of chants that could be employed. Thus, for cataract of the eye they used an instillation of isinglass and verdigris, accompanied by the chant: 'Come, verdigris! Come, verdigris! Come, thou Fresh One! Come, efflux from the eye of Horus! It comes, that which issues forth from the eye of Tum! Come, juice that gushes from Osiris!'

The Ebers Papyrus also contained a lengthy section on the diagnosis of illness, most of the diagnoses being concerned either with abdominal problems or with tumours. Thus, 'when thou examinest the obstruction in his abdomen and thou findest that he is not in a condition to leap the Nile, his stomach is swollen and his chest asthmatic, then say thou to him: "It is the blood that has got itself fixed and does not circulate."' There followed a remedy involving wormwood, elderberries, and beer, which 'remedy drives out blood through his mouth or rectum which resembles hog's blood when it is cooked.' And for a growth that 'comes-and-goes under thy fingers', and was thus probably a benign tumour, the quite appropriate treatment was excision: 'Treat it with a knife as one heals an open wound.'

Finally, the papyrus contained short sections on the hair, cosmetics, and household hints. A treatment which was said to encourage growth of hair on the balding scalp included the fat of lions, hippopotamuses, crocodiles, cats, serpents, and goats. While 'to drive away wrinkles from the features' a mixture of incense cake, wax, fresh olive oil ground together with fresh milk had to be applied to the face for six days. And finally, and very reasonably: 'To keep mice away from clothes—cat's fat, smear on everything possible.'

Clearly the papyrus contained some common-sense remedies, a lot of nonsense, and considerable amounts of magic and superstition. The great Greek physician Hippocrates (*c.* 460 to 380 BC) was vehemently opposed to such hocus-pocus. He maintained that a person's health depended upon a delicate balance of four body humours, blood, phlegm, black bile, and yellow bile, and that an imbalance of these produced illness. These beliefs were widely held until at least the time of Paracelsus (in the sixteenth century), but later physicians failed to appreciate Hippocrates' major contribution, which was that careful diagnosis was as important as appropriate prescribing. Hippocrates preferred to allow the patient to recover naturally with some minimal intervention using laxatives, purgatives, and emetics. His many medieval admirers were not so conservative.

Other Greeks made valuable contributions, notably Theophrastus (370 to 285 BC), whose classification of plants, entitled *Historia Plantarum*, was not bettered until the Renaissance, and of course Dioscorides. Owing to the decline of the Greek empire after the death of Alexander the Great (323 BC), all of the leading figures during the next few centuries were citizens of the Roman Empire. Pliny, Celsus, Scribonius Largus, and Dioscorides all wrote extensive treatises that included information on medicinal plants. Of these the eight volumes of *De Medicina* by Celsus included over 250 plant-derived remedies, and *De Materia Medica* by Dioscorides (AD 77) proved to be the most widely used through the centuries. The latter contained accounts of around 600 plants with advice on cultivation and harvesting as well as essential details of drug preparation and use. It was also beautifully illustrated in colour. Unfortunately most of the original works were lost during the barbarian invasions, and the oldest known Byzantine copy of Dioscorides' treatise forms part of what is known as the Juliana Anicia Codex (*c*. AD 512). The original Greek text was also translated into Arabic and Persian, thus forming a basis for later Moslem herbals, and the treatise was widely used in the west in the form of a Latin translation. In fact the famous herbals of Gerard and Culpeper incorporated and expanded upon the basic knowledge provided by Dioscorides.

As well as remedies from plants, the Greek Herbal contains advice on the use of living creatures and minerals. For example: 'Locusts being suffumigated, doe help the difficulties of pissing especially in women folke', and similarly 'grasshoppers if they be eaten roasted, doe help the griefs about the bladder'. While iron rust (*ios siderou*) 'doth stay ye woman's flux' and 'iron made burning hot, quenched in water, or wine, and drank, is good for ye coeliacall, dysentericall, splenicall, cholericall, and for a dissolved stomach'.

Galen (*c*. AD 129 to 199), another Greek, also left an indelible mark on the history of pharmacy. He studied anatomy and medicine for twelve years at Pergamum (his birthplace in Asia Minor), Smyrna, Corinth, and

Alexandria, then worked as a surgeon in the gladiatorial school in Pergamum, before moving to Rome. There he practised as a physician to the aristocracy and as a druggist. He carried out numerous anatomical and physiological experiments, and provided the first accurate information about the circulation of blood, the secretory functions of the kidneys, and the structure of the nervous system. These contributions were unrivalled until the Renaissance, but his pharmacy was less original. He based all of his numerous drug formulations on the Hippocratic theory of humours, and these vastly complex concoctions became known as galenicals. Given his reputation as a physician, his enthusiasm for this aberrant theory probably ensured its survival for another 1300 years.

The barbarian invasions heralded the Dark Ages in Europe (the fifth to eleventh centuries), and herbal knowledge was kept alive initially through the work of scribes in Constantinople, and then in the libraries of the rapidly expanding Arab empire. In China the Shên Nung herbal was updated, and a new eighteen volume herbal called *Nei Ching* appeared. In India the Hindu herbal of Susruta was published in the fifth century.

As the Arab empire spread eastwards towards India and westwards into Spain, a vast collection of mainly Greek books and manuscripts was amassed and eventually housed in a special library in Baghdad. Here, in the ninth century, a team of translators revised the earlier sixth century Syrian translations of Hippocrates, Dioscorides, Galen, and others, and produced new and more accurate versions in Arabic. The works of Galen were particularly popular, but the Arabs also had their own original writers on medicine and pharmacy. Prominent among these was Rhazes (*c.* 865–925) who embraced the ideas of Galen but was closer in his prescribing to the ideas of Hippocrates. His advice was: 'Where a cure can be obtained by diet use no drugs, and avoid complex remedies when simple ones will suffice.' He also demonstrated the probable toxicity of many of the popular remedies based on heavy metal salts, especially those involving mercury, by using his pet monkey as a test animal.

Rhazes was followed by Avicenna (930–1036), probably the most influential Islamic writer of the age, and like Rhazes a skilled alchemist, physician, and pharmacist. His main work was entitled *A Canon on Medicine*, and in it he followed the doctrines of Galen and Hippocrates in assuming the importance of the four humours. In the book he provided information on drugs, compound medicines, and diseases of various parts of the body; but this compilation was later overshadowed by the comprehensive *Corpus of Simples* by Ibn al-Baitar (1197–1248) of Malaga. This contained a list of 1400 drugs and medicinal plants, mostly derived from the works of Dioscorides and Far Eastern herbals.

Meanwhile, during the Dark Ages in Europe, pharmacy, superstition, and magic became inextricably intertwined. A number of 'leechbooks' (from the Anglo-Saxon *laece*, to heal) were compiled, containing some recognizable drugs, but mostly fanciful brews for fending off elves and goblins. The most famous of these leechbooks is undoubtedly the *Leechbook of Bald*. Bald was probably a friend of Alfred the Great, and the book dates from about 900–950, which makes it the oldest surviving Saxon book on herbal use. It certainly incorporates herb lore from earlier centuries, but the original works were destroyed when the Vikings sacked the monasteries. Even a cursory examination of this leechbook leaves one in no doubt that Bald and his contemporaries believed explicitly in the existence of elves and goblins. According to Bald, disease was primarily due to 'elf-shot' or 'flying venom', and his herbal brews were both protective and curative. For protection against the elfin peril: 'A salve against the elfin race and nocturnal goblin visitors: take wormwood, lupin . . . Put these worts into a vessel, set them under the altar, sing over them nine masses, boil them in butter and sheep's grease, add much holy salt, strain through a cloth. . .' And a cure for a cold: 'Take nettles, and seeth them in oil, smear and rub all thy body therewith; the cold will depart away.'

Monastic medicine became pre-eminent from around the tenth century, though the various Church Councils (1131–1212) eventually forbade the monks from participating in medical practices. Their extensive libraries became the repositories of herbal knowledge and a number of comprehensive treatises appeared. The most famous of these were the *De Viribus Herbarum*, usually attributed to Odo, Bishop of Meung (the medicinal properties of eighty plants were described in Latin verse), the *Antidotarium* of Nicolaus of Salerno (in reality a collective work on medicinal plants from the active school of medicine in Salerno), and the *Liber de Proprietatibus Rerum* of Bartholomaeus Anglicus, an English professor of theology in Magdeburg This last encyclopaedic work first appeared in around 1260, and it included descriptions of medicinal plants along with information on angels and demons, the body's essences, winged creatures, meteorology, cosmology, geography, and much, much more. It was a kind of thirteenth century *Encyclopaedia Britannica* in nineteen sections. In the herbal section he wrote (of the mandrake): 'The rind thereof medled with wine . . . geve to them to drink that shall be cut in their body for they should slepe and not fele the sore knitting.' This is very reminiscent of similar remedies prescribed by Dioscorides and mentioned in Chapter 1.

The great medical schools in Salerno and Montpellier were a source of most of the information on pharmacy during the thirteenth and fourteenth centuries, and during this period the freelance apothecaries began to ply their trade. These were originally known as pepperers and spicers (*pévriers* and *épiciers* on the Continent), and they dealt in drugs, potions, and perfumes. The arrival of the printing press in the fifteenth century allowed these apothecaries to gain access to the works of Galen, Dioscorides, and Theophrastus, and to the recently compiled *Grand Herbier*. This appeared in the late 1480s and ran to nearly 500 chapters. It subsequently formed the basis of the first important English herbal, which was published by Richard Bankes in 1525. This is still medieval in character and the prose is charming. For example, the virtues of rosemary are comprehensively surveyed: 'Take the flowers and put them in thy chest among thy clothes or among thy Bookes and Mothes shall not destroy them'; and 'If thy legges be blowen with gowte boyle the leave in water and binde them in a linnen cloath and winde it about thy legges and it shall do thee much good.'

A greater reputation was accorded to *The Grete Herball* published by Peter Treveris in 1526, though this contains many strange remedies. For example: 'To make folke mery at ye table, take foure rotes of vervayne in wyne, then spryncle the wyne all about ye house where the eatynge is and they shall be all mery.' But other plant extracts, including liquorice, laudanum, and olive oil, were certainly efficacious.

An altogether more scientific text was the *New Herball* of William Turner, which appeared in parts between 1551 and 1562, and then as a whole (dedicated to Elizabeth I) in 1568. He was educated at Cambridge and published a little book, the *Libellus de Re Herbaria Novus*, in 1538, followed ten years later by a handbook of medicinal plant names in Greek, Latin, English, Dutch, and French. This was sorely needed, because the level of botanical knowledge in England at that time was abysmal. His fiercely nonconformist views soon brought him into conflict with the Crown, and he spent two years in jail before a period of exile in Europe. His books were also destroyed. During his exile he gathered information for the herbal, the first part of which was published (in 1551) during the more tolerant reign of Edward VI. A second period of exile and the destruction of most copies of the herbal ensued during the short reign of Mary I, but he returned to favour and to publish other parts of the herbal in the reign of Elizabeth.

The *New Herball* can be considered as the first true British Flora, with over 200 native species included, and it contained botanical and herbal information. Of mandrake he wrote: 'If mandragora be taken out of measure by and by slepe ensueth and a great lousing of the streyngthe with a forgetfulness.' And for an overdose of opium: 'If the pacient be to much slepi put stynkynge thynges unto hys nose to waken hym therewith.'

If William Turner is the 'father of English botany', then Paracelsus (the sobriquet of Theophrastus Bombastus von Hohenheim) is the 'father of European pharmacy and pharmaceutical chemistry'. He was born near Zurich in 1493 and trained to be a physician in Italy, though most of his knowledge is claimed to have originated from his dealings with gypsies and midwives. He was appointed professor of medicine and city physician of Basle in 1527, and almost immediately created a sensation by publicly burning the works of Galen and Avicenna. He was particularly scornful of their complex herbal remedies and was a firm believer in magic and the 'doctrine of signatures'. This ancient belief claimed that the shape of a plant determined its utility, as with the mandrake's human form and its use as a treatment for infertility. He is mainly famous for his alchemy and his use of metal salts as remedies, in particular for syphilis, but his plant drugs were also widely used. His tincture of opium, which he christened 'laudanum', was especially popular.

Several European herbals appeared during this period, but most of these were based upon the works of Galen and Dioscorides, and provided little new knowledge of pharmacy. Peter Schoeffer's *Herbarius Latinus* (Mainz, 1484) was primarily concerned with medieval German plant lore, e.g. 'coriander taken with vinegar soon after dining heavily prohibits vapours rising to the head'. While Jacob Meydenbach's *Hortus Sanitas* (Mainz, 1491) comprised 1066 chapters and 1073 illustrations with numerous highly imaginative prescriptions. For example, the magnetic lodestone was claimed as a diagnostic aid to establish fidelity: 'When this stone is placed beneath the head of a faithful woman, she is . . . moved to open her arms to her husband . . . Yet if she be an adultress then through evil dreams she will suffer much fear and trembling.' The effect upon an unfaithful husband is not revealed.

These herbals appeared at the time of Christopher Columbus's momentous voyages of discovery, and not surprisingly the ones that appeared in the sixteenth century incorporated information on the newly discovered plants. Foremost among these was the *Dos libros* of Nicholas Monardes (Seville, 1569), which contained descriptions of tobacco, coca, sarsaparilla, etc. This was reprinted in English by John Frampton in 1579 under the title *Joyfull Newes out of the Newe Founde Worlde*. Medicinal plants from the other side of the world were described by Garcia d'Orta, onetime physician in Goa, under the title *Coloquios dos simples, e drogas e cousas medicinais da India* (Goa, 1563), and several later editions appeared in Latin, English, Italian, and French. But pride of place in any list of fifteenth century herbals must go to John Gerard's *The Herball, or Generall Historie of Plantes*.

John Gerard (1546–1612) was certainly well acquainted with medicinal plants, since for twenty years he cared for the gardens of Lord Burghley, Secretary of State under Elizabeth I, and in addition had his own physic garden off Chancery Lane in London. In the 1590s he was asked to assist with a translation of a Belgian herbal entitled *Pemptades* by Rembert Dodoens, and it seems that he made changes and rearrangements of the text in order to pass off the translated work as his own. The result was a very flawed text with numerous errors, and the eminent botanist Mathias

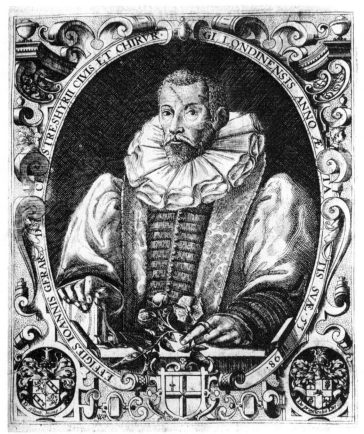

John Gerard, author of *The Herball, or Generall Historie of Plantes* (1598). (Wellcome Institute Library, London.)

de l'Obel (after whom the genus *Lobelia* is named) was called in to help rectify this problem. The ultimate work published in 1597 was thus very much a joint effort, though Gerard's name is always associated with the *Herball*. His main contributions were in the sections on English flora and their uses, and these are described in near poetic fashion. Two examples will suffice for the present. Of the newly introduced tobacco he wrote: 'The drie leaves are used to be taken in a pipe set on fire and suckt into the stomacke, and thrust forth again at the nostrils against the paines of the head, rheumes, aches in any part of the bodie.' And of the dwarf water lily: 'The flowers being made into oile . . . doth coole and refrigerate, causing sweat and quiet sleepe, and putteth away all venereous dreames.' With 1392 pages of text and 2821 woodcuts the book remains a monumental and very readable treatise.

None of the aforementioned herbalists was a practising apothecary, and at least in England many of the apothecaries had turned to alchemy in the sixteenth century, leaving much of the prescribing to charlatans. These specialized in ointments, plasters, and lotions, made with salts of arsenic and mercury, for the treatment of syphilis. For centuries the apothecaries had been part of the Grocers' Company, but in 1617 the apothecaries resident in London formed themselves into a corporate body called the Worshipful Society of the Art and Mystery of Apothecaries. The seventeenth century thus saw the beginnings of a more ordered system for the prescribing of drugs, and the first *London Pharmacopoeia* appeared in 1618. This contained a list of 1190 'simples' (remedies consisting of a single drug). During the seventeenth century, a genuine apothecary would have served a seven-year apprenticeship, during which he would have learnt how to prepare and dispense all manner of medicines. They often practised as physicians and even surgeons as well. Two such apothecaries were John Parkinson (1567–1650) and Thomas Johnson (1604–1644). The former was 'herbarist' to Charles I, and had his own apothecary shop in Long Acre, London. His best known work is the *Theatrum Botanicum*, or the *Universall and Compleate Herball*, published in 1640. This ran to 1755 pages and was highly detailed. Thomas Johnson is mainly remembered for his extensive revision of Gerard's *Herball*, which now contained 2850 descriptions of plants. No doubt he would have left a greater legacy had he not been actively involved in the Civil War: he died as a result of wounds received while defending Basing House in Hampshire.

Nicholas Culpeper (1616–1654) also fought (and was wounded) in the Civil War, but on the side of the Parliamentarians. Unlike the other two he never completed his apprenticeship as an apothecary, but he did obtain a medical qualification and practised as a physician and astrologer. He wrote many books, but he will always be remembered for his herbal *The English Physician Enlarged, with 369 Medicines made of English Herbs* published in 1653. This was widely read and used until the nineteenth century. Of senna he wrote: 'It is under the dominion of mercury . . . it is of a purging faculty, but leaveth a binding quality after the purging . . . it purgeth melancholy, choler, and phlegm, from the head and brain, lungs, heart, liver, and spleen, cleansing those parts of evil humours . . . it strengthens the senses and procureth mirth . . . [it] works very violently both upwards and downwards, offending the stomach and bowels.' The astrological interest is apparent throughout the treatise, and of hemlock he wrote: 'Saturn claims dominion over this herb, yet I wonder why it may not be applied to the privities in a priapism, or continual standing of the yard, it being very beneficial to that disease.'

Further editions of the *London Pharmacopoeia* appeared in 1621, 1623, 1639, and 1650, but these still contained a preponderance of remedies based upon the use of inorganic salts. These included *mercurius sublimatus corrosivus* (mercuric chloride), *regulus antimonii* (metallic antimony), and *plumbi lotio* (dilute lead acetate solution), not to mention 'prepared worms and millipedes'. The other major publishing event (in 1657) was the apothecary Richard Tomlinson's translation of the *Dispensatory* of Jean de Renou, a physician at the French court, whose book was the first true book of pharmacy and pharmaceutical practice. In it he described such techniques as infusion, decoction, and humectation, and his list of preparations included numerous gargles, pessaries, lotions, and linaments. As usual, tried and tested plant extracts like senna, aloes, and rhubarb appear with inorganic remedies like mercury and yellow arsenic, and other highly dubious 'drugs' like rubies, lodestone, foxes' lungs, and dog's dung.

This confused state of pharmaceutical practice persisted for some time in England, because, unlike their foreign counterparts, the English universities had no departments of pharmacy. However, many university chemists and botanists seem to have had an interest in pharmacy, and Robert Boyle's *The Skeptical Chymist* published in 1661, laid the foundations for an understanding of the chemistry of drugs. The old ideas of Aristotle concerning the four elements (earth, air, fire, and water) were finally swept away, and a chemical element was defined as a substance that could not be broken down into simpler substances.

'Chymists' and druggists were now often one and the same, and several English pharmaceutical companies had their origins in this epoch. For example, Allen & Hanburys (now part of the Glaxo Group) can trace its origins to the apothecary Sylvanus Bean, who set up shop in Old Plough Court in London in 1715. These eighteenth century apothecaries were importers of large amounts of raw materials, which were converted into such widely used preparations as tincture of Peruvian bark (for malaria) and cod liver oil (for rheumatism and rickets).

Williams Withering's *An Account of the Foxglove and some of its Medical Uses* appeared in 1785. It was the first thoroughly scientific account of the use of a folk medicine, and it showed how a careful evaluation of patients' case histories could provide information about the correct dosages and routes of administration for the efficacious use of herbal remedies.

Major advances in chemical knowledge occurred at the end of the eighteenth and beginning of the nineteenth centuries, and the newer techniques allowed the isolation of purer drugs from natural sources. The *London Pharmacopoeia* of 1809 mentioned the use of aconite, belladonna, cinchona, colchicum, hemlock, henbane, and opium, and constituent alkaloids of these and other medicinal plants were isolated soon after: morphine (1816), strychnine from seeds of *Nux vomica* (1817), atropine (1819), quinine (1820), and colchicine (1820).

The numerous small companies that were set up in the late nineteenth century, specializing in these plant extracts and in fine chemicals, were the forerunners of the modern pharmaceutical industry. The German company Bayer was the first to commercialize (in 1899) a synthetic drug based upon a herbal remedy, aspirin, and this is still the largest selling drug of all. However, it is worth noting that most of the pharmaceutical companies originally made their fortunes from inorganic preparations, for example, Beechams' liver pills (bismuth salts) and Boots' Epsom salts (basically magnesium sulphate). The era of drug discovery based upon naturally occurring substances and herbal remedies did not begin until well into the twentieth century. These triumphs of chemistry and pharmacology are the subject of the rest of this book.

Antibacterial substances

Folk remedies for the treatment of wounds, boils, burns, and other conditions liable to bacterial infection, or caused by infection, abound in the ancient treatises. For example, the Ebers papyrus includes preparations based upon raw meat (for the bite of a crocodile), goat's dung and fermenting yeast (for a burn), scribe's excrement and fresh milk (for boils), and oil and honey (for an ear infection). This last remedy would have at least been soothing, but the subsequent treatment involved an extract of gazelle's ears, tortoise shell, and the annek plant.

Three thousand years later Ambroise Paré, a noted army surgeon and subsequently surgeon to the French King Henry III, extolled the virtues of a mixture of new-born puppies boiled in oil of lilies, earthworms, and Venetian turpentine as a treatment for gunshot wounds. This was, in fact, Paré's speciality, and other healing remedies used the medicinal herbs sage, rosemary, thyme, camomile, lavender, and melilot, together with red roses boiled in white wine, oak ashes, and a little vinegar.

Other plants that were reputed to contain antibacterial substances included hops, garlic, wild ginger, the common wallflower (the seeds were said to be especially good for mouth ulcers), pumpkin, aloes, dock, and sorrel. Gerard and Culpeper recommended numerous concoctions. From Gerard: 'The fruite (of the Balsam apple, *Tanacetum balsamita*) . . . boiled in a double glass set in hot water, or else buried in horse dung; taketh away inflammations that are in wounds.' And from Culpeper: '[Goldenrod, *Verbascum thapsus*] is a sovereign wound herb inferior to none, both for the inward and outward hurts.'

Numerous healers used poultices prepared from mouldy bread or soil, and as with all of the other remedies mentioned these probably had little efficacy and usually exacerbated the condition of the infected wound. There was almost total ignorance of the nature of infection until the pioneering studies of Pasteur and Koch in the middle of the nineteenth century.

When the microscope was invented by Antony van Leeuwenhoek in the 1670s, it became possible for the first time to view microorganisms, or 'animalcules' as he termed them. His letters reveal his excitement upon first seeing these 'creatures': '. . . the number of these animalcules was so extraordinarily great . . . that 'twould take a thousand million of some of 'em to make up the bulk of a coarse sand-grain . . .'.

A proper scientific study of these microorganisms was impossible until it was realized that contamination of bacterial and fungal cultures by other bacteria or fungi was the norm rather than the exception. Without the means to sterilize equipment and to work under aseptic conditions, pure colonies of microorganisms could not be prepared. The advance of microbial knowledge was also retarded, because it was heretical to suppose that microorganisms appeared other than by divine intervention, that is by spontaneous generation. For centuries it had been the general belief that moulds appeared spontaneously upon decomposing matter. These ideas were finally refuted through the careful experiments of Spallanzani in the eighteenth century, who demonstrated that boiled meat would remain free of contaminants provided that it was kept properly covered. Schwann repeated these experiments in 1837 and further showed that even if air was allowed to reach the meat no putrefaction occurred as long as the air was heated (to destroy microorganisms).

But it was the elegant experiments of Pasteur that provided the firm basis of microbiological knowledge which made possible the formulation of a germ theory of disease. Pasteur was educated as a chemist and spent much of his early career investigating the nature of fermentation. He demonstrated that certain microorganisms (yeasts) mediated alcoholic fermentation, while others (lactobacilli) controlled the fermentation of milk products. Through these studies he established the ubiquity of the various organisms, especially in the soil.

Historically there were a number of theories about the spread of infection. Galen believed that epidemics were caused by 'miasmas' or poisonous vapours produced whenever the conjunction of the planets was unfavourable. Fracastorius (of Verona) spoke in his text *De Contagion* (1746) of 'seminaria' or seeds of contagion. Edward Jenner in 1796 observed that milkmaids rarely contracted smallpox, and thus used material from pustules of the cowpox (a similar, though less virulent, viral disease) as a vaccination against smallpox. However, the implications of this prophylactic procedure were not apparent to him.

The first demonstration of the communicability of disease was carried out by John Snow in 1854, who traced the source of an isolated cholera epidemic in London to a contaminated water pump in Broad Street. Later, Joseph Lister was sufficiently impressed by Pasteur's demonstration of the ubiquity of microorganisms to initiate the use of antisepsis in his surgical operations and in the recovery wards.

In 1865, when Lister first introduced carbolic acid (phenol) as an antiseptic, mortality following amputations was round 50 per cent, and on the battlefield it was probably closer to 100 per cent. Natural phenolic substances had been used for centuries as preservatives, as in the ancient Egyptian embalming mixtures, but one of the problems facing Lister was the refusal by his hospital staff to accept that wounds became contaminated by airborne (or more often surgeon-borne) pathogens. As early as 1835 the American physician Oliver Wendell Holmes had shown that the incidence of puerperal fever (caused by post-natal bacterial infection) could be dramatically reduced if hands were washed with chlorine-based disinfectants. The Hungarian physician Ignaz Semmelweis and the Scot Alexander Gordon confirmed this finding and managed to reduce the mortality from puerperal sepsis in the wards from above 10 per cent to around 1 per cent.

Lister tried carbolic acid, because it had proved useful in a national campaign to eradicate the putrefying effects of microorganisms in sewers. Other phenols, like salicylic acid and guiacol (from creosote), were later used both externally and internally, and it was during attempts to identify less corrosive antiseptics that Fleming discovered lysozyme and then penicillin.

Before those momentous discoveries, the German country physician Robert Koch made several significant contributions. He demonstrated that anthrax bacilli isolated from dead sheep could be transmitted to healthy animals. Koch and other German investigators subsequently isolated the causative organisms for tuberculosis, cholera, typhoid, diphtheria, and tetanus, as well as various types of bacteria, including streptococci, pneumococci, meningococci, and staphylococci. These investigations paved the way for the discovery of the antibiotics.

It is often forgotten that life expectancy at the beginning of the Victorian era was a mere 45 years, and that infant mortality in England remained doggedly at around 150 per thousand live births throughout the nineteenth century. It was common for a trifling infection to become life-threatening, and during the great flu pandemic of 1918–19, twenty million people died, mainly from pneumonia, a bacteria-induced complication of a primary viral infection. This figure is far larger than the number of casualties which resulted from the Great War of 1914–18.

The original concept of one microorganism killing another, so-called 'antibiosis', was introduced by Pasteur in 1877, when he showed that the growth of anthrax bacilli in urine could be prevented by the addition of several common bacteria. He confirmed this result using animals, and similar results were obtained by Freudenreich (1888) and Nicolle (1907). The latter carried out particularly thorough experiments with *Bacillus subtilis*, in which extracts from this organism were used to inhibit the growth of the bacteria that caused typhoid, cholera, and pneumonia. But it was Sir John Burdon-Sanderson who first demonstrated that certain *Penicillium* moulds would prevent the growth of bacteria in culture.

Lister was convinced that the mould *P. glaucum* could be used to treat humans, and in 1884 he treated a young nurse, Ellen Jones, who had a large, non-healing abscess. She received topical applications of the mould extract and made a good recovery. Several other people worked with what was probably the bacterium *Penicillium brevicompactum*, and demonstrated its antibacterial properties, but none of these investigators pursued these interesting discoveries.

During World War I Alexander Fleming worked as a bacteriologist in a hospital near Boulogne, and was particularly involved with those casualties whose wounds involved complex bone fractures, which were especially susceptible to complications involving gas gangrene. When the flu pandemic struck in 1918–19, the hospital was inundated with patients suffering from pneumonia, and Fleming took numerous bacteriological samples for analysis. His main finding was that the virus seemed to weaken the lungs and render them susceptible to infection with any of the common bacteria, streptococci, staphylococci, etc., and the previously fit young men and women ultimately died of asphyxiation, drowning in their pulmonary exudate.

On his return to England Fleming took up a post at St Mary's Hospital in Paddington, and during 1921 he studied the bacteriolytic agents present in human secretions, e.g. in tears and nasal mucus. Unfortunately most of these preparations were not particularly active and the secretions were not easily available. A famous *Punch* cartoon of the time showed a drill sergeant beating a small boy, whose tears were then collected in a bottle marked 'tear antiseptic'. This was inspired by Fleming's use of boy volunteers, who donated tears after the instillation of lemon juice into their eyes.

This practice ceased once egg white had been identified as a better source of the main bacteriolytic agent, christened lysozyme, and Fleming and his co-workers continued with their painstaking efforts to explore the efficacy of lysozyme against various bacteria. The value of this pre-

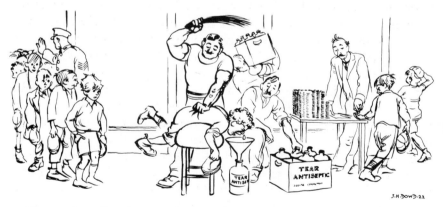

Cartoon from *Punch* (1922) by J. H. Dowd depicting the collection of 'tear antiseptic'. In reality, the boys had lemon juice instilled into their eyes, and the resultant tears were collected. (Reproduced by kind permission of Punch Publications Ltd., London.)

penicillin work is often overlooked, but without the expertise and knowledge gained during these years it is doubtful whether Fleming would have realized the significance of his discovery in September 1928.

In his paper in the *British Journal of Experimental Pathology* of 1929, Fleming stated quite baldly that some cultures of staphylococcus had been left on the open bench, and after contamination with an airborne mould 'it was noticed that around a large colony of a contaminating mould the staphylococcus colonies became transparent and were obviously undergoing lysis'. This description fails to reveal the quite extraordinary chain of chance events that allowed the discovery to be made.

Firstly Fleming left a pile of used culture plates containing staphylococci on the end of a bench while he went away on holiday. During his absence a relatively rare strain of *Penicillum* came in through the window (presumably) and contaminated one of the plates. Initially the weather was cool, thus favouring growth of the *Penicillum* mould, but later in the month there was a warm spell and this favoured growth of the bacteria. On his return Fleming piled the plates into a shallow tray containing the disinfectant lysol, before cleaning them properly, but the key plate was (fortuitously) not immersed. He was examining this pile of plates more or less at

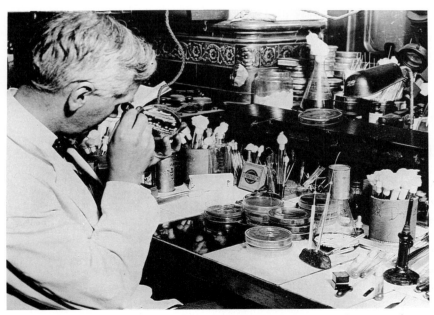

Alexander Fleming in his laboratory at St Mary's Hospital. (From the photographic archives, St Mary's Hospital, Paddington.)

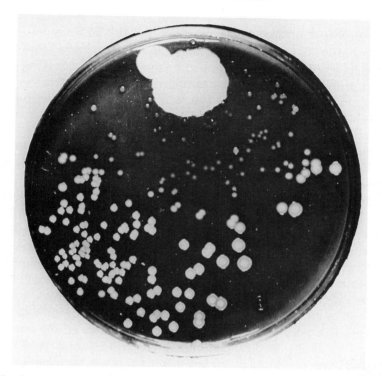

The famous culture plate. The mould is at the top. Note that there is no bacterial growth in the vicinity of the mould. (From the photographic archives, St Mary's Hospital, Paddington.)

random, when he spotted one with a blob of mould and an absence of staphylococcal colonies around it.

His co-workers were unimpressed, but Fleming propagated the mould and in due course demonstrated that extracts of the mould would inhibit the growth of streptococci, staphylococci, pneumococci, meningococci, gonococci, and diphtheria bacilli. This meant that it was much more broad-spectrum in its activity than lysozyme, and on a par with the strongest antiseptics. Once it had been identified as a *Penicillium*, Fleming christened the extract (hitherto known as 'mould juice') 'penicillin'. The actual strain of mould was finally identified in 1929 (as *Penicillium notatum*) by Charles Thom, an American mycologist who was to play a leading part in the later scaling-up of penicillin production.

Fleming got two of his graduate assistants, Frederick Ridley and Stuart Craddock, to grow larger quantities of the mould in order to obtain sufficient penicillin for further biological evaluation. They found that the mould grew best at room temperature and provided an optimum yield of penicillin after about ten days. Concentration of the extract had to be effected under reduced pressure and at a temperature not exceeding 40 °C, and the product was soluble in ethanol, which implied that it was not a protein. The resultant penicillin had high antibacterial activity but was only stable under near neutral conditions (pH around 6.5) and for at most two to three weeks.

In vivo experiments showed that the biological lifetime of penicillin was very short and also confirmed its serious acid instability. This somewhat diminished the chances of therapeutic utility, but Fleming none the less tried the extract on several human guinea-pigs, including Craddock (who had a chronic nasal infection) and an amputee with early signs of septicaemia. The latter subsequently died and the former was hardly improved, but eventually they recorded a success. One of the laboratory assistants, K. B. Rogers, was due to compete in an important shooting competition but contracted pneumococcal conjunctivitis. Instillation of penicillin into his eyes effected a complete cure and the world could have had the beginnings of an antibiotic revolution there and then, but for the fact that Fleming was a poor public speaker. When he announced the results of their studies at the Medical Research Club on 13 February 1929, his lecture was very poor, and the audience failed to realize the significance of the discovery. Fleming's seminal paper in the May issue of the *Journal of Experimental Pathology* also went largely unheeded, and it took a further twelve years before the potential of penicillins was realized.

What probably counted against Fleming most of all was that others had already described the antibacterial activity of *Penicillium* moulds, so his work seemed relatively unoriginal. It was the high potency of Fleming's strain that made it special, as well as the sheer serendipity of the chain of events that had led to its discovery. Fortunately the group at St Mary's propagated their mould continuously during the next decade, primarily because it was used to kill bacteria that interfered with the growth of laboratory specimens of *Haemophilus influenzae*. This ensured that the mould was available when Florey's group in Oxford began to study penicillins.

Howard Florey, an Australian by birth, was educated at Adelaide Medical School and then held a postgraduate scholarship at Oxford University, followed by a research studentship at Cambridge, and then a year in America. He was appointed a lecturer in the Pathology Department at Cambridge University in 1927 and began a study of the properties of lysozyme, so much of his work paralleled that of Fleming. In 1930 he

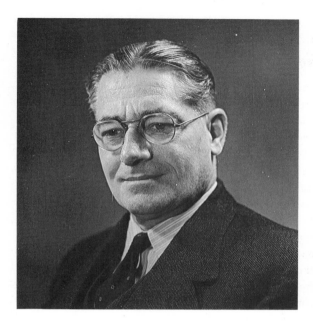

Howard Florey (c. 1941), Professor of Pathology at the Sir William Dunn School of Pathology, University of Oxford (1935–62). (Reproduced by kind permission of the Sir William Dunn School of Pathology.)

reported the actual lysozyme content of saliva, tears, and various other secretions of the goat, guinea-pig, rat, and rabbit.

In March 1932 he was appointed professor of pathology at Sheffield University, and among other research projects he developed (with H. E. Harding) a treatment for tetanus that involved the administration of curare in conjunction with artificial ventilation of the patient. The principles of this treatment are still used in cases of tetanus. Another missed opportunity occurred during Florey's time at Sheffield, and this also involved the pathologist H. E. Harding, who informed Florey that a colleague, G. C. Paine, had cured a pneumococcal infection in a patient's eye by using 'mould juice' obtained from a culture of Fleming's strain of *Penicillium*. Florey apparently registered no interest in this discovery, which of course exactly replicated the cure achieved by the St Mary's group.

In 1935 Florey moved to the newly endowed Chair of Pathology at the Sir William Dunn School of Pathology in Oxford and set about attracting a team of bright, young research workers. Lysozyme was still the main topic of research, and Ernst Chain, a Jewish refugee from Nazi Germany, finally elucidated its mode of action in 1937. He showed that in susceptible bacteria it would cleave the polysaccharides of their cell walls, thus initiating disintegration of the cells.

A more comprehensive search for antibacterial substances was initiated in 1938, and among the organisms investigated was the strain of *Penicil-lium notatum* that had been maintained by Fleming's group since 1929. Chain (a biochemist) and E. P. Abraham (a chemist) duplicated much of the previous work on the isolation and purification of penicillin, and their colleague Norman Heatley managed to improve the technology dramati-cally. They passed crude, slightly acidic 'mould juice' against a counter-current of the solvent amyl acetate, and the amyl acetate extract was then passed against a countercurrent of slightly alkaline water. The aqueous extract was then freeze-dried to produce a brown powder which possessed relatively high antibacterial activity, although it was subsequently shown to contain only around 0.1 per cent active penicillin and 99.9 per cent impurities.

On 25 May 1940, eight mice infected with a lethal dose of streptococci were used for an *in vivo* experiment. Three were given multiple doses of penicillin, one was given one dose, and the remainder were given no penicillin at all. The first three mice survived while the other five died. Further experiments confirmed these results, and for the first time the exciting antibacterial potential of penicillin was revealed. It is a sobering thought that the amounts of crude penicillin Florey and his group used were probably similar to those used by Fleming twelve years earlier, but the latter failed to grasp the significance of his work.

However, the dawn of the era of antibiotics was to be delayed still further, because these crucial experiments were taking place while the British Expeditionary Force was being evacuated from Dunkirk. In fact, the Oxford group were so worried about the likelihood of a German invasion that they deliberately contaminated their clothing with spores of *Penicillium notatum* and determined to escape to America with their precious discovery.

The task was now to produce large quantities of penicillin for a human trial, and since no pharmaceutical company could be persuaded to partici-pate, Florey and his co-workers undertook the job themselves. They had already experimented with various kinds of vessels for growth of the mould, including trays, pie dishes, and hospital bedpans. The latter proved to be particularly effective, so they grew the mould in 600 specially commissioned bed-pan-shaped pottery vessels, and used dairy equipment for a much-improved extraction process. Chromatography on alumina*

---

*Alumina chromatography is a purification technique which uses the differential partition of chemical compounds between a moving solvent phase and the aluminium oxide adsorbent, in order to effect a separation of the compounds.

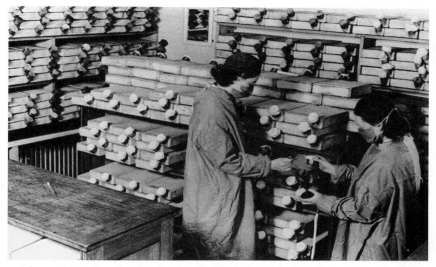

The penicillin 'production line' at the Sir William Dunn School of Pathology (c. 1940). The mould was grown in the ceramic vessels and dairy equipment was used for the extraction and purification stages. (Reproduced by kind permission of the Sir William Dunn School of Pathology.)

also afforded a greater degree of purification, and by the middle of January 1941 they had enough material for a clinical trial.

Initially they injected the drug into a terminally ill cancer patient (a Mrs Elva Akers of Oxford) with no ill effects, and then into healthy volunteers, thus establishing the correct dose rate to maintain a bacteriostatic effect. Finally, six patients, all with life-threatening bacterial infections, were treated between February and June and the case histories as well as a full account of the growth, harvesting, and purification of 'penicillin' were reported in the *Lancet* of 16 August 1941.

The first patient was a 43-year-old policeman, Albert Alexander, who had developed a generalized infection with *Staphylococcus aureus* and *Streptococcus pyogenes* after suffering a facial scratch from a rosebush. By the time treatment started he had lost one eye and had numerous abscesses on his face and on one arm. There was also evidence of lung damage. On 12 February he was given 200 mg of penicillin, followed by further injections of 100 mg at two- to four-hourly intervals for five days. His condition improved dramatically, and by 17 February his temperature was normal, he was eating well, and most of the infections showed signs of healing. The supplies of penicillin were so limited, even allowing for the quantities recovered from his urine, that his treatment was discontinued so that another seriously ill patient could be treated. In the event they exhausted all of their available penicillin on the second patient and had none left to treat Alexander when he suddenly relapsed ten days later. He died on 15 March from staphylococcal septicaemia.

The tragic outcome of this first treatment was not repeated with the second patient, a boy of 15 who had contracted streptococcal septicaemia after a hip operation. He received a total of 3.4 g of penicillin over a five-day period and went on to make a complete recovery.

By May fresh supplies of penicillin were available and a 48-year-old labourer with a four-inch carbuncle and evidence of further spread of staphylococcal infection was successfully treated. His complete recovery within seven days was nothing short of miraculous for such a condition. Then came a second tragedy. A 4½-year-old boy was admitted to the Radcliffe Infirmary with an infection in the base of his brain. This had originated from infected measles spots on his face and left eyelid. At the time of admission he was semi-comatose and had grossly swollen eyelids.

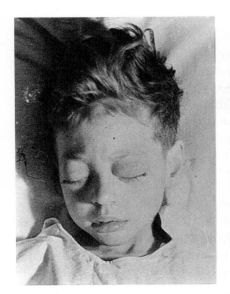 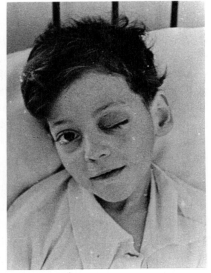

Before and after treatment with penicillin. This 4½ year old boy was treated with penicillin and made a dramatic recovery from a bacterial infection caused by measles. Tragically, he later died of a brain haemorrhage caused by damage to blood vessels in the early stages of his infection. (Reproduced by kind permission of the Sir William Dunn School of Pathology.)

He received penicillin continuously from 13 May to 25 May, during which time he made a dramatic recovery: the swelling was much reduced, his temperature was normal, and he began playing with toys and talking to the hospital staff. But, as with the policeman, he suddenly relapsed and died of a brain haemorrhage. A post-mortem examination showed that the bacterial infection had been completely eradicated by the penicillin, but that during the initial stages of the infection, irreversible physical damage had been suffered by several cranial blood vessels. This was another tragic conclusion, but as Florey and co-workers noted: 'Before this vascular accident the patient had been restored from a moribund condition to apparent convalescence.'

The other two cases—one a 14-year-old boy with septicaemia, the other a baby with an acute urinary infection—were completely cured with penicillin, as were four less serious cases of acute eye infections. The paper in the *Lancet* concluded with the statement: 'Enough evidence, we consider, has now been assembled to show that penicillin is a new and effective type of chemotherapeutic agent, and possesses some properties unknown in any antibacterial substance hitherto described.' With this rather modest statement they announced the dawn of the antibiotic era.

The pharmaceutical industry was none the less slow to appreciate the potential value of these results, though their resources were already heavily committed to the war effort. Fleming now re-entered the arena and reminded the medical world that it was he who had recognized in his 1929 paper the potential of penicillin. This aroused not a little interest in the popular press: for example, the once popular weekly picture magazine *Titbits* ran a story about 'The Cure that Came in the Window'. Many of the myths about Fleming's discovery originate from this time.

Unable to scale up their process any further, Florey sought industrial help in the USA, and the Bureau of Agricultural Chemistry at Peoria, Illinois, took on the task of executing a commercial-scale fermentation. They improved the culture medium by using corn-steep liquor (a waste product from corn starch production), and America's entry into the war in December 1941 ensured a total dedication to a project that would ultimately benefit their battlefield casualties.

Florey was forced back to the Dunn School and the bedpans for his own supplies of penicillin, although small amounts were produced by ICI and a small London company called Kemball-Bishop. During 1942 the Oxford group treated 187 patients, and a mere handful failed to respond completely. Even Fleming became involved when a friend of the family, Harry Lambert, became seriously ill with meningitis. Florey provided the penicillin and Fleming injected it, intravenously at first, but then intrathecally (directly into the subarachnoid space in the brain) when he discovered that the penicillin was not gaining entry to the brain. Despite the fact that this route of administration had never been used before, the patient made a rapid recovery, and Fleming was finally persuaded of the importance of the new antibiotic.

His direct approach to friends within the Government led to the establishment of the Penicillin Committee, and thence to the involvement of companies like ICI, Glaxo, and Burroughs Wellcome, who were soon producing tens of millions of units of penicillin every month. This, however, paled almost into insignificance when considered alongside the 100 000 million units per month being produced by the American companies Merck, Squibb, and Pfizer by the middle of 1944. This massive improvement in yield was made possible by the use of a new strain of mould, *Penicillium chrysogenum*, and through the use of deep fermentation tanks similar to those used in the brewing industry. The new strain came originally from a mouldy canteloupe found in the market at Peoria.

The American public was largely unaware of these momentous events, though there was a flurry of publicity when the wife of the Yale University Director of Athletics, Mrs Ogden Miller, was cured of a life-threatening streptococcal septicaemia in March 1942. But little news leaked out after the very successful use of penicillin to treat the many victims of a fire at the Coconut Grove nightclub in Boston in January 1943.

Florey spent the rest of the war years involved with clinical trials of penicillin, especially in relation to the treatment of war wounds. Through this work he discovered that gonorrhoea could be completely cured within twelve hours of administration of penicillin. This was of considerable value, since at that time in North Africa there were more VD sufferers than wounded. During these same war years Fleming and Florey were involved in acrimonious exchanges, since the British press had accepted Fleming as the sole inventor of penicillin, a misconception which remains in some people's minds to this day, despite the awarding of the Nobel prize in physiology and medicine jointly to Fleming, Florey, and Chain in 1945.

After the end of the war the structure of the major penicillin produced by *Penicillium chrysogenum*, so-called penicillin G, was elucidated by Dorothy Hodgkin using X-ray crystallography, and chemical synthesis was attempted. John Sheehan of the Massachusetts Institute of Technology was the first to devise a practical route to 6-aminopenicillanic acid, a major building block of the penicillins, and this then allowed the construction of other novel semi-synthetic penicillins.

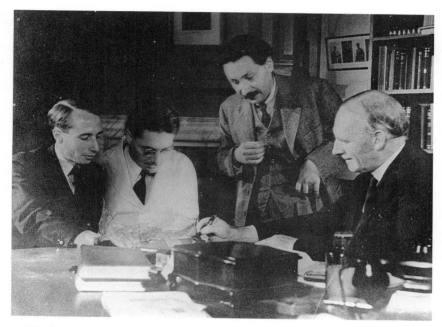

Working on the structure of penicillin. From left to right: Edward Abraham, Wilson Baker, Ernest Chain, and Robert Robinson (c. 1945). (Reproduced by Kind permission of the Sir William Dunn School of Pathology.)

In addition, Beechams had discovered that 6-aminopenicillanic acid was actually a stable product present in the fermentation mixture, and could be isolated and converted into novel penicillins, while Eli Lilly in the USA discovered that addition of side-chain precursors (of the desired penicillin structures) to the fermentation brew enhanced production of the corresponding penicillins. This allowed the introduction of the relatively acid-stable penicillin V (phenoxymethylpenicillin) in the mid-1950s, and since this could be given orally (rather than by injection) it allowed GPs to prescribe the drug for home use.

Other semi-synthetic penicillins followed in rapid succession, with an increasing emphasis on broad-spectrum antibacterial activity (i.e. activity against a wide range of bacteria) and acid stability. With the ready availability of these antibiotics there was a degree of over-prescribing by GPs, but more importantly they were incorporated into animal feeds on a massive scale. This meant that the bacteria were forced to evolve a means of resistance or become extinct, and since a bacterium will typically reproduce itself every twenty minutes or so, the time-scale for the evolution of resistant strains is a much faster process than with other organisms.

By the early 1960s most strains of bacteria had developed at least some degree of resistance to penicillins, achieving this through the development of specialized enzymes (β-lactamases) that cleave part of the penicillin structure, thus rendering penicillins inactive. In order to understand the mechanism of this process it is necessary to understand how the penicillins exert their antibacterial activity.

All of the bacteria which are susceptible to the penicillins, the so-called Gram-positive species (because they can be dyed with the Gram stain), have a cell wall with a structure comprising polysaccharide chains linked to polypeptide chains cross-linked in an overall three-dimensional lattice. When the bacterial cell divides, it needs to produce new cell wall material, and it does this by converting a two-dimensional polysaccharide–polypeptide structure into the three-dimensional cross-linked structure of the cell wall. The mechanism of this process is shown in Fig. 4.1, and in outline this simply involves cleavage of the terminal amino acid (an alanine) from one polypeptide chain and coupling of the penultimate amino acid (also an alanine) on to the terminal amino acid (usually a glycine) of a polypeptide side-chain. Penicillin functions through inhibition of the enzyme involved in this process, a transpeptidase. This enzyme is 'fooled' by the similarity in shape between the antibiotic and the last two amino acids (alanine–alanine) of the polypeptide chain (see Fig. 4.2) and reacts with the antibiotic, becoming essentially inextricably bound up with it and thus unavailable for the cross-linking operation.

The β-lactamases of resistant bacteria attack the four-membered ring of the penicillins (the β-lactam ring) and break it open, thus preventing its reaction with the transpeptidase enzyme. Cell-wall construction can then proceed unimpeded. Recently, a number of pharmaceutical companies have introduced β-lactamase inhibitors. These are not necessarily antibacterial, but they do prevent the β-lactamases from damaging the penicillins. One recent drug combination from Beechams is particularly interesting, since this combines a broad-spectrum penicillin (amoxycillin) with a naturally occurring inhibitor of β-lactamases (clavulanic acid).

Aside from the problem of resistance, a number of other difficulties arose during the clinical application of penicillins. First, a small proportion of the population were found to be allergic to the drugs. Second, most penicillins were not active against Gram-negative bacteria like *Salmonella* and *Pseudomonas*. These organisms are especially prevalent in developing countries, where they cause debilitating infections, and they are also

Polysaccharide chain

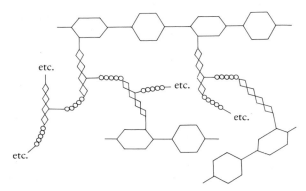

A — Transpeptidase cleaves a terminal alamine

B — The three-dimensional cell wall matrix after cross-linking

Fig. 4.1 Mechanism of action of penicillin.

especially dangerous for patients whose immune system has been compromised, like those undergoing cancer chemotherapy or (more recently) those suffering from AIDS.

The work on the penicillins stimulated others to search for moulds that had antibacterial activity, and in 1948 Giuseppe Brotzu set in train a series of events that were almost as exciting as those initiated by Fleming twenty years previously. He was the director of the Istituto d'Igiene in Cagliari, Sardinia, and had isolated a mould, taken from the vicinity of a sewer outlet, which inhibited the growth of typhus bacilli. This was significant because penicillin was not active against such Gram-negative organisms. He effected a partial purification and used his crude extract in the successful treatment of patients with boils and abscesses caused by Gram-positive organisms, and even obtained some success in patients suffering from typhoid and paratyphoid. However, the Italian authorities showed no

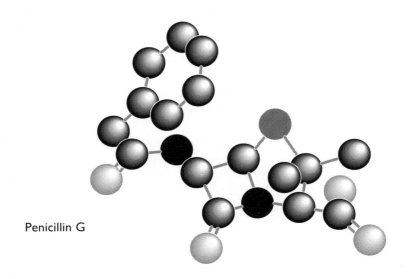

Penicillin G

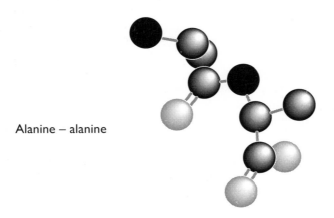

Alanine – alanine

Fig. 4.2 Comparison of the structures of penicillin G and alanine–alanine.

interest in his work, and in desperation Brotzu contacted a friend who had earlier been Public Health Officer in Cagliari. He in turn arranged for Florey to receive a culture of the mould.

The mould was identified as *Cephalosporium acremonium*, and the William Dunn School swung into action once more to investigate and exploit its antibacterial activity. After several false starts the team led by E. P. Abraham isolated a weak antibacterial substance, and this they christened cephalosphorin C. It had two advantages over penicillin G— very low toxicity and resistance to β-lactamases—but the introduction of methicillin by Beechams in 1960, which was also resistant, seemed to diminish the prospects for cephalosporin C. These were revived following the discovery by Eli Lilly that the basic structural skeleton of penicillin G could be chemically transformed into that of cephalosporin C, and a whole array of novel cephalosprins was then synthesized.

The present situation is that the cephalosporins, unlike the penicillins, have proved generally resistant to attack by β-lactamases and also have a broader spectrum of activity than the penicillins. However, they are more expensive to produce and so, although products like cephaclor and cepha- lexin are widely prescribed orally active cephalosporins, most of the newer drugs are reserved for hospital use. And the search goes on for novel synthetic and naturally occurring antibiotics.

Soil microorganisms have always proved to be repositories of interest- ing natural products, especially antibacterial substances, and contempor- aneous with the studies of Chain and Florey, Selman Waksman began a screening programme with vast numbers of soil microorganisms. His prime aim was to find a substance that would inhibit the growth of *Mycobacterium tuberculosis*, the causative agent of TB. In 1943 he and his co-workers finally isolated streptomycin from *Streptomyces griseus*, and this was effective not only against *M. tuberculosis* but also against a whole range of other pathogens. In the clinic it was a great success, though a major adverse effect was deafness through irreversible damage to the auditory nerve.

Other soil microorganisms soon revealed their secrets. These included chloramphenicol (from *Streptomyces venezuela*), now usually reserved for severe conditions like meningitis and for topical use in infections of the eyes and ears, the tetracyclines (from various *Streptomyces*), which were the first semi-synthetic, orally active antibiotics in the early 1950s, and griseofulvin (from *Penicillium griseofulvum*), which was first isolated in 1939 and which subsequently proved to be especially efficacious against fungal infections (e.g. ringworm) in cattle and humans. Many others have proved to be effective anticancer agents.

So although the efficacy of mouldy bread poultices and soil plasters is dubious, moulds and soil microorganisms have provided a rich source of valuable antibacterial and antifungal agents. These drugs have made a major contribution to increased longevity and quality of life in the twentieth century. Like most other modern drugs, they were products of the combined efforts of chemists, biochemists, pharmacologists, and clinicians.

Anti-inflammatory agents

The leaves [of comfrey] bruised with the white of an egg, and applied to any place burnt with fire, takes out the fire, gives sudden ease, and heals it up afterwards.

This remedy from Culpeper neatly summarizes the symptoms of inflammation: warmth and reddening, pain, swelling, and associated tissue damage. There are two main types of inflammatory state: chronic and acute. The former includes such conditions as rheumatoid arthritis, rheumatic fever, psoriasis, and emphysema, while the latter includes hay fever and sunburn. These all involve a response by the tissues to an irritant of some kind. Commonly the tissue affected is in the lungs or respiratory tract (e.g. emphysema and hay fever), joints (e.g. rheumatoid arthritis), or skin (e.g. psoriasis and sunburn).

Many of the chronic inflammatory conditions are the result of so-called autoimmune diseases, which, as the term suggests, implies that the sufferer produces antibodies which destroy his or her own tissues. A good example of this is provided by rheumatic fever, in which an infection with a haemolytic streptococcus induces the production of antibodies that destroy not only the invading pathogen but also, in genetically predisposed individuals, heart (valve) tissues, producing an inflammatory state. In rheumatoid arthritis the autoantibodies are directed against the joints, and cellular destruction leads to the production of hydrolytic enzymes that initiate further damage and the symptoms of chronic inflammation.

The primary causes of acute inflammation are mechanical or chemical damage, radiation (e.g. heat, ultraviolet, or radioactive), and foreign organisms (e.g. bacteria, fungi, pollen, or parasites). The chemical mediators of the classic symptoms of warmth and reddening, pain, and swelling (easily visualized as the sequel to excessive exposure to the sun) include histamine, kinins (small peptides), eicosanoids (all derivatives of the fatty acid arachidonic acid), and in some tissues 5-hydroxytryptamine (also called serotonin). All of these, especially histamine, are potent mediators of vasodilation, i.e. they induce a widening of the blood vessels. As the inflammatory state takes hold, blood platelets and leukocytes may aggregate near the site of damage to form a clot or thrombus. The pain results from a stimulation of local nerve-endings by histamine, serotonin, or the kinins.

The mediators mentioned above originate primarily (though not exclusively) from the white blood cells known as mast cells, and a typical sequence of events that precedes the release of these substances is depicted in Fig. 4.3. This shows the interaction of an allergen (e.g. ragweed pollen, house dust mites, etc.) with antibodies specific for these substances that are bound to the surface of the mast cells. These antibodies of the immunoglobulin E (IgE) class are produced in much greater amounts by persons who have a genetic disposition to allergy and asthma. The formation of

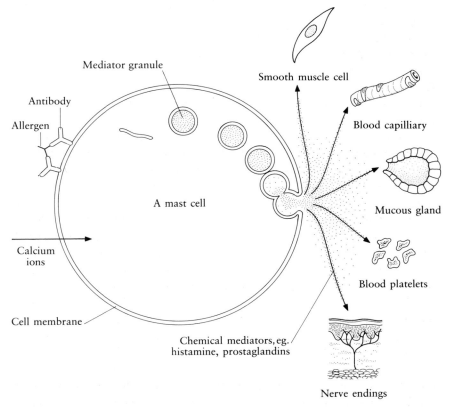

Fig. 4.3 The mast cell and its involvement in inflammation.

this antibody—allergen complex results in a change of shape of the mast cell surface and the opening of 'gates' over calcium channels. The resultant in-rush of calcium ions leads to an activation of a number of cytoplasmic enzymes which catalyse the formation of histamine and eicosanoids. The cell eventually ruptures, and these substances are released and interact with other cells, precipitating the acute inflammatory states associated with allergy, such as asthma, eczema, and hayfever. It is interesting to note that hayfever and other allergies appear to have increased in incidence during the last two centuries, and this is probably linked to the rapid rise in environmental pollution during the same period.

Numerous additional kinds of cellular interactions are implicated in the inflammatory state, and these involve other chemical mediators, such as the kinins, but also more exotic species like lymphokines, platelet activating factor, tissue necrosis factor, etc. Although a complete understanding of these processes is still a long way off, we can derive a very reasonable idea of the modes of actions of the known anti-inflammatory drugs by considering their interactions with the system shown in Fig. 4.3.

There are innumerable remedies listed in the various herbals, and most plants have found favour at one time or another. In the Ebers papyrus the treatments for inflammatory conditions include onion crushed in honey and taken in beer, chopped bat in a poultice, wasp's dung and fresh milk, or a piece of lead in admixture with cat's and dog's dung applied as a poultice.

Dioscorides recommended (amongst other plants) coriander (*Coriandrum sativum*): '[It] is well known, having a facility of cooling, whence being applied with bread . . . it heals ye *Erysipelata* (St Anthony's fire) and creeping ulcers.' This belief was confirmed by Gerard: 'The juice of the leaves mixed and laboured in a leaden mortar, with ceruse, litharge of silver, vinegar and oile of roses, cureth St Anthony's fire, and taketh away all inflammations whatsoever.' He was even more enthusiastic about the thorn-apple (*Datura stramonium*): 'The juice of thornapples boiled with hogges grease to form an unguent or salve, cureth all inflammations whatsoever, all manner of burnings or scaldings, as well of fire, water, boiling lead, gunpowder . . .'.

Culpeper was especially keen on wintergreen (*Gaultheria procumbens*): 'Wintergreen is under the dominion of Saturn, and is a singularly good wound herb . . . a salve made of the green herb stamped, or the juice boiled with hog's lard . . . is a sovereign salve, and highly extolled by the Germans, who use it to heal all manner of wounds and sores.' He also recommended burdock, camomile, comfrey, feverfew, goldenrod, hyssop, rue, and hemlock. Of the latter he wrote: 'It may be safely applied to inflammations, tumours, and swellings in any part of the body, save the privy parts.'

The North American Indians never produced a herbal, but much of their folk medicine has been recorded by Virgil J. Vogel in his book entitled *American Indian Medicine*, and it is clear from this that witch-hazel (*Hamamelis virginiana*) was the plant most often prescribed for inflammations. This was obviously efficacious, because as recently as 1965 the Eli Lilly catalogue included a proprietary medicine containing witch-hazel, thorn-apple, and other ingredients that was 'a soothing, palliative ointment for temporary relief of the pain of haemorrhoids.' The witch-hazel provided the anti-inflammatory action and the hyoscine from the thorn-apple acted as a local anaesthetic.

Most of the herbals also mentioned extracts of willow leaves or bark as a treatment for inflammation, and these were chosen because the ancients believed that remedies were usually located in places where a disease was most prevalent. Thus, rheumatic complaints were common in damp places where the willow thrived. The Ebers papyrus contains a particularly apposite description of both the inflammatory condition and the efficacy of willow extracts:

When you examine a man with an irregular wound ... and that wound is inflamed ... [there is] a concentration of heat; the lips of that wound are reddened and that man is hot in consequence ... Then you must make cooling substances for him to draw the heat out ... leaves of the willow.

Gerard recommended the leaves and bark of willows to 'staye the spitting of blood, and all other fluxes of the blood', while Culpeper recommended them for another kind of 'inflammation': 'The leaves bruised and boiled in wine, and drank, stays the heat of lust in man or woman, and quite extinguishes it, if it be long used.'

In the seventeenth and eighteenth centuries cinchona bark (which contains quinine) was the most popular remedy for treating internal inflammatory conditions, and the first report of the use of willow extracts, given by the Reverend Edward Stone, did not appear until the end of the eighteenth century. He treated patients with the ague (i.e. fever, usually meaning malaria) with 20 grains (about 1 g) of powdered willow bark in a dram of water every four hours, and claimed favourable responses.

The first proper clinical trial was carried out in 1876 by the Scottish physician Thomas MacLagan, who treated 100 patients suffering from rheumatic fever. He administered salicylic acid, which was obtained by chemical transformation of salicin, the major active constituent extracted from willow bark. His treatment resulted in complete remission of the fever and joint inflammation that is characteristic of this disease. Some six years earlier Professor Marcellus von Neuki of Basel had shown that salicin was converted *in vivo* into salicylic acid and, with others, had demonstrated the efficacy of this compound in lowering the temperatures of patients suffering from typhoid and rheumatic fever.

A factory at Dresden was set up to satisfy a world-wide demand for salicylic acid and also its sodium salt, but though the treatment of febrile conditions was highly successful the large doses administered were not only unpleasant tasting but also caused gastric irritation and damage. This was largely overcome by the introduction of acetylsalicylic acid by the German company Bayer in 1899. They christened this 'aspirin', the name originating from the 'a' of acetyl and the 'spir' of *Spirea ulmania*, the plant from which salicylic acid had originally been isolated. Bayer registered this tradename, and an intense wrangle then ensued between Bayer and other German companies that sold acetylsalicylic acid. Bayer argued that if a physician prescribed aspirin, their product must be dispensed. The pharmacist could only dispense other forms of acetylsalicylic acid if the prescription called for *Ersatz für Aspirin*.

At the end of World War I Bayer lost their exclusive right to the name aspirin, when the allies sequestrated their property. During the war the allies had mounted a major competition to devise an alternative chemical route for the synthesis of aspirin, and the prize of £20 000 was eventually won by an Australian, George Nicholas, who called his product 'Aspro'.

Acetylsalicylic acid is still the most widely used drug, and in excess of 25 million kilograms are produced annually. The daily consumption figures in the USA (*c.* 35 000 kg) and the UK (*c.* 6000 kg) provide cogent evidence of its popularity as an antipyretic (temperature-lowering), analgesic, and antirheumatic drug. The major adverse effect of its long-term use is gastric ulceration, although the risk of this can be reduced through the use of soluble forms of aspirin.

Elucidation of its mode of action was something of a milestone in pharmacology. In 1971 John Vane and his co-workers at the Wellcome Foundation showed that it inhibited one of the key enzymes involved in the production of prostanoids (prostaglandins, thromboxanes, and prostacyclin). These are all members of the family of chemical compounds known as eicosanoids and are all produced from arachidonic acid (eicosatetraenoic acid). These prostanoids are produced in microgram amounts by many cells, and are required for the control of normal bronchiolar function, the control of gastric acidity, the induction of labour at full-term of pregnancy, the control of blood platelet aggregation, etc. They also act as mediators of inflammation, bronchoconstriction, pain, and fever.

Aspirin inhibits the key enzyme cyclo-oxygenase and prevents the formation of the prostanoids, but it fails to inhibit other enzymes known as lipoxygenases, which control the formation of other classes of eicosanoids— the leukotrienes, lipoxins, etc. These are also mediators of inflammation and have a key role in asthma and allergy. It is thus clear why aspirin can alleviate at least some of the symptoms of an inflammatory episode and also why it causes problems in the gut.

More recently it has been suggested that aspirin and the other non-steroidal anti-inflammatory drugs (NSAIDs, described below) also modify the functions of the white cells known as neutrophils. These are major participants in the body's defence against invasion by foreign organisms, allergens, etc., and are also implicated in the various autoimmune diseases. They damage cells by releasing proteases which destroy proteins, and also through the release of highly reactive forms of oxygen, like peroxide and superoxide. The NSAIDs appear to prevent aggregation of neutrophils and adhesion of neutrophils to other cells, both of which are necessary for tissue damage. Further research will be required before the mechanisms of action of aspirin and the other NSAIDs are fully understood.

The newer anti-inflammatory drugs have been designed to combine the useful analgesic, antipyretic, and anti-inflammatory properties of aspirin with a reduced level of gastric toxicity. Typical of the drug modification experiments were those carried out by Boots Ltd, involving the synthesis of numerous structural analogues of aspirin. As so often happens, their first active compound (Boots 7268) had originally been prepared for agricultural use (as a potential weedkiller), but it was twice as potent as aspirin when tested in an anti-inflammatory screen. About 600 similar compounds were prepared, and the most active (Boots 8402) was six to ten times more potent than aspirin. Further structural manipulation led ultimately to the highly effective drug ibuprofen (Brufen and Nurofen), which was not only up to thirty times more potent as an anti-inflammatory agent but also possessed good analgesic and antipyretic properties (thirty times and twenty times greater than aspirin respectively). This drug has proved to be both effective and safe over long periods of use, and it is now available as a non-prescription item in many countries.

Other pharmaceutical companies have made similar discoveries, and naproxen (Naprosyn), from Syntex, is also widely used. Both of these drugs are members of the group of compounds known as non-steroidal anti-inflammatory drugs (NSAIDs), and the name reveals that the other important class of anti-inflammatory agents are steroids.

It has probably been known for hundreds of years that women suffering from rheumatoid arthritis experience a major amelioration of their symptoms if they become pregnant. The first suggestion that this might be due to the actions of a hormone was made by the physician Philip Hensch in 1930, and he christened this putative substance 'compound E'. The identity and source of the hormone were not established until the 1940s, when it was shown to be the steroid cortisone which is produced by the adrenal glands (Fig. 4.4), where it is synthesized from cholesterol.

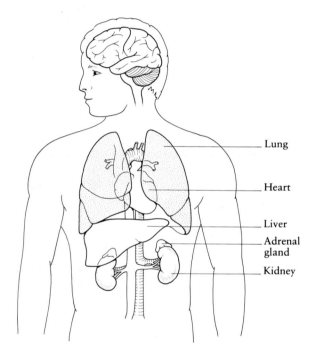

Fig. 4.4 The main organs of the human body.

Cholesterol is the main mammalian steroid, and a human adult typically contains about 250 g of this compound. Some of this is obtained from the diet, but the majority is manufactured in the liver. Much of this cholesterol is involved as a constituent of cell membranes or is converted into bile acids, which assist with the assimilation of fats from the diet. Very tiny amounts are used for the construction of the steroid hormones: the corticosteroids in the adrenals and the sex hormones in the ovaries or testes.

The first group of hormones includes the anti-inflammatory steroids, which will be discussed in this section. The latter class will be considered in the section on the reproductive system.

Production of the corticosteroids is under the control of the hypothalamus, a small area in the central part of the brain. This releases a number of peptides, which in turn stimulate the release of specific peptide hormones from the pituitary. Corticosteroid synthesis in the adrenals is initiated by one of these hormones, ACTH (adrenocorticotrophic hormone), and two types of steroid are produced: the glucocorticoids and the mineralocorticoids. The latter are primarily concerned with the regulation of mineral balance (especially of sodium and potassium ions) and fluid balance.

The glucocorticoids, notably cortisone and hydrocortisone, stimulate the production of glucose, especially in the liver, and promote its conversion into its polymeric storage form, glycogen. To do this they can mobilize protein from muscle and degrade it to produce amino acids, which can then be used as 'building blocks' for glucose production (glucogenesis). Release of the glucocorticoids is stimulated if one is placed under stress, and the resultant increase in metabolic activity helps us to survive such stressful environmental changes.

In 1948 cortisone (still known as compound E) was available as the product of a thirty-six-stage industrial chemical synthesis, but not surprisingly supplies were limited, and 1 g of the drug cost about $200. Hensch obtained enough of the drug to treat one patient who was desperately ill with rheumatoid arthritis, and she made a dramatic (if temporary) recovery, with almost complete alleviation of pain and reduction in the swelling in her joints.

As a result of this clinical trial a major effort was initiated by the pharmaceutical industry to produce large quantities of this 'miracle drug'. G. D. Searle embarked upon a large-scale extraction of cortisone from cattle adrenal glands, while Syntex investigated the chemical conversion of the female hormone progesterone into cortisone and structural analogues. They already had a good supply of progesterone, thanks to the pioneering efforts of Russell Marker, who had identified several steroid-containing plants and had then used these steroids as starting materials for the synthesis of progesterone. The full story of this discovery and its relevance to the invention of the contraceptive steroids will be described in the section on the reproductive system.

In addition, the Upjohn Company was also involved in the quest for cortisone, and they ultimately succeeded through using the fungus *Rhizopus nigricans*. They effected a biochemical conversion of progesterone (10 tons were supplied by Syntex at 48¢ per gram) into 11-hydroxyprogesterone and then by chemical manipulation into hydrocortisone.

However, although both drugs were very effective anti-inflammatory agents, they also possessed significant mineralocorticoid activity. This meant that patients suffered from potentially dangerous disturbance of their fluid, sodium, and potassium balance, and the drugs are now mainly reserved for local use and are injected directly into the affected joints of arthritis sufferers.

Despite this set-back, the pharmaceutical industry had a lead compound, and in the ensuing forty years numerous structural analogues of these natural steroids have been prepared and evaluated. Much of the work has been carried out by Syntex in the USA and Glaxo in the UK and has relied on the original idea of Russell Marker of obtaining precursor steroids from plants. Syntex initially obtained their precursor (diosgenin) from a Mexican plant of the *Dioscorea* genus, but subsequently discovered that hecogenin from the American agave, *Agave sisalina*, was a better starting material. In 1951 Syntex reported the synthesis of cortisone from hecogenin and subsequently licensed their process for use by Glaxo. The latter improved on the Syntex route, and both companies commercialized their processes and produced a number of therapeutically useful drugs. Of these fluocinolone acetonide (Synalar, Syntex) and betamethasone valerate (Betnovate, Glaxo) are probably the best known and most widely prescribed for topical use, e.g. for the treatment of eczema and psoriasis. For internal (systemic) use, the most commonly prescribed anti-inflammatory steroid is still prednisolone, though in recent years there have been some remarkable advances in the design of steroids for the treatment of asthma. As will become clear in the section on the respiratory tract, an asthmatic attack, whatever its cause, is the most prominent manifestation of an underlying inflammatory state in the lungs. In an attempt to treat this chronic condition, Glaxo introduced beclomethasone dipropionate (Becotide) which is administered as an aerosol using an inhaler. In doses of 300–400 micrograms per day there was no significant effect on systemic steroid metabolism (i.e. no effects on mineral balance or on hormonal status), and the drug has been very effective in controlling the symptoms of asthma in a large number of sufferers. It is also used as a nasal spray for alleviating the misery of hay fever.

The mode of action of these anti-inflammatory steroids is still largely a mystery. They are believed to stabilize certain organelles (storage vessels) within mast cells, thus preventing the release of histamine and the enzymes involves in the production of prostanoids. In addition, they probably inhibit the production of collagenase enzymes, which are involved in destruction of connective tissue.

Clearly there is still much to be learnt about inflammation and the modes of action of the drugs that are used to treat the various inflammatory conditions. None the less it is pertinent to note that most of the advances described in this section have occurred since 1948, and we will not celebrate the centenary of the introduction of aspirin until 1999.

Drugs affecting the reproductive system

Most of the functions and malfunctions of the human body described so far in this chapter are largely beyond the control of mere mortals, but with sexual reproduction there is at least the opportunity to exercise some control. Not surprisingly people have had a long-term interest in plant extracts that control fertility, induce abortion or labour depending upon the period since conception, or possess aphrodisiac activity.

Of the herbalists Culpeper seems to have had the greatest interest in this area, and it comes as no surprise that the plants he recommended were all under the control of Venus. Of tansy (*Tanacetum vulgare*) he wrote: 'Dame Venus was minded to pleasure women with child by this herb . . . This herb bruised and applied to the navel, stays miscarriages . . . Let those women that desire children love this herb, it is their best companion, their husbands excepted.' He went further, claiming that 'the very smell of it [tansy] stays abortion or miscarriages'. The plant feverfew was no less effective: 'Venus commands this herb, and has commanded it to succour her sisters and to be a general strengthener of their wombs.' For those who liked to take their herbs with alcohol, 'a decoction of the flowers in wine, with a little nutmeg or mace put therein, and drank often in a day, is an approved remedy to bring down women's courses speedily'.

Whatever the effects of these herbal brews, most of the physiology and biochemistry of reproduction is under the control of the steroidal sex hormones. These are produced in response to the release by the pituitary of peptide hormones: luteinizing hormone (LH) and follicle stimulating hormone (FSH), the so-called gonadotrophins. In the female these act upon the ovaries to stimulate production of oestrogens, which leads in turn to changes in the reproductive tract and the production of progesterone. In the male the gonadotrophins act upon the testes and stimulate the production of androgens like testosterone.

Small amounts of these hormones are produced from birth, but their concentrations rise dramatically at puberty and initiate the development of secondary sexual characteristics: beard growth and deepening of the voice in men, and growth of the mammary glands in females. More generally they lead to the observed differences between the sexes in the distribution of hair and body fat, and in body build consequent upon changes in the skeleton and muscles. Perhaps most important of all, subtle changes in the concentrations of female hormones are responsible for the menstrual cycle and for maintenance of pregnancy after conception.

Between puberty and the menopause, a period of around thirty to forty years, an ovum is prepared each month for possible fertilization. Under the influence of LH and FSH, one or more small cells (follicles) that contain immature ova begin to develop in the ovary. As the follicle grows it begins to secrete oestrogens, and these in turn act upon the surface layer of cells in the uterus, the endometrium, causing it to thicken. About three days before ovulation there is a surge in the concentrations of oestrogens and LH, and this induces release of the mature ovum. Yet another pituitary hormone, prolactin, is now released and acts upon the ruptured follicle causing it to produce progesterone and small amounts of oestrogens. These hormones act upon the endometrium preparing it for the reception of a fertilized ovum, and also exert a 'feedback' inhibition on the pituitary, preventing further release of LH or FSH. If fertilization does not occur, the concentrations of progesterone and oestrogens fall, the corpus luteum breaks up, and the lining of the endometrium is shed, resulting in menstruation. A summary of the cyclical changes of hormone concentrations and their consequences is depicted in Fig. 4.5.

If fertilization occurs, the blastocyst (fusion of sperm and ovum) embeds itself in the wall of the uterus and secretes the hormone human chorionic gonadotrophin. This functions rather like LH and inhibits the destruction of the corpus luteum, which responds with increased amounts of progesterone and oestrogens. These initiate fresh growth of the endometrium and there is, of course, no menstruation. The menstrual cycle also ceases because the continual production of high concentrations of progesterone by the corpus luteum, and also by the developing placenta, suppresses the release of LH and FSH.

In the past these early signs of pregnancy would often have induced the 'sufferer' to seek a plant-derived abortifacient from a quack or herbalist. Dioscorides recommended 'abortion wine': 'Amongst ye vines there is planted *Veratrum*, or wild cucumber, or scamone, of which ye grape doth take the faculty, and the wine made of them becomes destructive [of the fetus]. It is given with water ... to women fasted, having first vomited.' The Shoshoni Indians also used a decoction made from the roots of

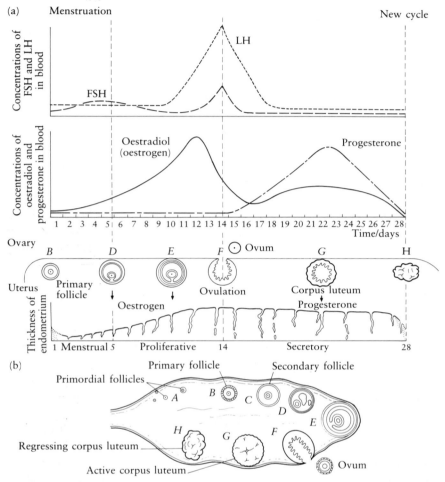

Fig. 4.5 The menstrual cycle. A section through the human ovary showing the cellular changes during the cycle.

Veratrum californicum, but as a contraceptive rather than as an abortifacient. But the most successful herbal contraceptive was undoubtedly the tea made from leaves of the Mexican plant zoapatle (*Montana tomentosa*). This could induce menstruation or labour, and certainly regulated fertility. Recent research by the Ortho Pharmaceutical Corporation has demonstrated the efficacy of the major constituent, zoapatanol. This and a range of synthetic analogues prevent conception or cause early abortion if administered to guinea-pigs, but no human trials have as yet been carried out.

Fertility control on a massive scale and with a high degree of reliability was made possible by the discovery of the contraceptive 'pill'. This arose out of a desire to find a drug that would prevent spontaneous abortion (miscarriage) rather than one that would exert control over fertility. During the period 1929–35 many of the steroidal sex hormones were isolated in pure form, though they were always in short supply. This is hardly surprising when one realizes that to obtain 12 mg of the oestrogen oestradiol, it was necessary to extract 4 tons of sow ovaries. None the less, in 1934 enough progesterone was available to allow its administration to women who habitually miscarried. The hormone was very effective, but its expense precluded large-scale trials.

Synthetic work by the chemist Ruzicka in Switzerland culminated in 1937 in the production of ethisterone, an orally active progestational agent (progestogen), and the related drug ethinyl oestradiol, which had good oestrogenic activity. The latter is still the agent of choice for hormone replacement therapy (HRT). This is given to women after the menopause to help reduce the changes in mood that often accompany the loss of female hormones. It also helps to reduce the incidence of brittle bone disease, which is again due to the diminished concentrations of oestrogens and associated changes in calcium metabolism.

In 1950 George Pincus, of the Worcester Foundation for Experimental Biology, and John Rock, a gynaecologist at Harvard University, designed the first oral contraceptive based on a regimen of progesterone for three weeks followed by withdrawal of the drug for one week to allow menstruation to occur. However, the dosages of drug were high (about 300 mg daily), and about one in five women experienced incomplete control of their cycles, with resultant 'breakthrough bleeding'. Clearly a more potent progestogen was required.

For the solution to this problem one has to recall the work of the steroid chemist Russell Marker (mentioned briefly in the section on anti-inflammatory drugs). In 1939 he was attempting to identify a cheap and renewable source of steroid hormones. His idea was to use natural plant sterols and to carry out a chemical conversion of these compounds to the hormones. Initially he worked with sarsasapogenin from sarsaparilla root, but in 1940 he turned his attentions to diosgenin, from *Dioscorea* species. He devised an efficient chemical route from diosgenin to progesterone and then scoured the south-western states of the USA and Mexico for a good source of diosgenin. Eventually he found a local species in the state of

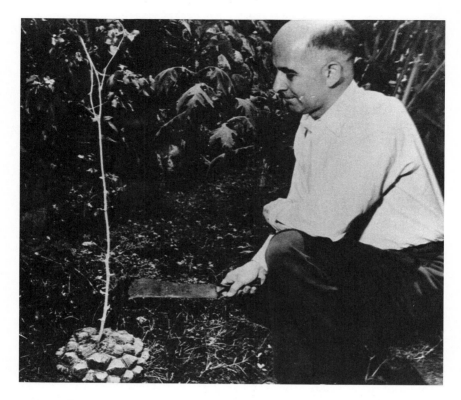

Russell Marker with a specimen of *Dioscorea*, taken in the early 1950s. Marker's major contribution was his development of a route to relatively large quantities of progesterone from the natural product diosgenin found in the plant. (Reproduced by kind permission of the Pennsylvania State University Archives.)

Veracruz, which contained large quantities of his starting material, and, having failed to interest the US pharmaceutical industry in his ideas, he set up his own laboratory in Mexico City and went into production.

According to legend he appeared one day in 1943 in the offices of a local drug marketing company, Laboratorios Hormona, with around 2 kg of progesterone wrapped up in old newspapers. This was worth about $160 000 at the time and represented a sizeable proportion of the annual production of progesterone. The outcome of this remarkable event was the founding of the drug company Syntex, and Marker went on to prepare several more kilograms of progesterone before leaving the company in

1945 after a disagreement. His successor, George Rozenkranz, had received his research training with Ruzicka and used his knowledge of steroid chemistry to devise or improve routes from diosgenin to all four classes of steroid hormones: androgens, oestrogens, progestogens, and corticoids. Of these, the oestrogens were the most challenging targets, because they possessed a very different structure from the other hormones. However, with the able assistance of the American chemist Carl Djerassi, destined to become president of Syntex, the problem was solved in 1950.

By 1951 they had prepared a novel progestogen called norethisterone (Norethindrone), while the Searle Company had also produced a structurally similar compound known as norethynodrel. Both of these compounds proved to be effective progestogens, and a large-scale clinical trial began in Puerto Rico in 1956. Each of 221 women received norethynodrel and 1–2 per cent of a synthetic oestrogen (mestranol) in the form of tablets (Enavid) during a two-year period, and only those who withdrew from the trial became pregnant. After a further study involving 1600 women Searle was given permission to market the first oral contraceptive in 1960.

Numerous other formulations were tried over the next fifteen years, and the relatively high dosage of progestogen used at the outset (about 10 mg daily) was soon shown to be unnecessary. Syntex's highly effective Norinyl was launched in 1964 and contained 2 mg of norethindrone and 0.1 mg of mestranol. At the end of the decade fears over the oestrogen content of the pill were aroused when it was noted that there was a higher than normal incidence of heart attack and stroke in women who were long-term users of the pill. As a result most oral contraceptives now contain tiny amounts of oestrogen in conjunction with small amounts of progestogens. It is of interest that the long-term use of progestogens has recently been shown to have a significant preventive action against breast cancer.

As to the mode of action of these contraceptives, it is now clear that the main effects of the progestogen are twofold. It causes changes in the cervical mucus, which becomes thicker, thus impeding the progress of the spermatozoa, and the endometrium suffers changes that render it less favourable for implantation. The drugs thus provides what Dioscorides could not: a means by which a woman can control her fertility with confidence and the minimum of fuss.

The herbalists paid scant attention to the control of male fertility, though the Chinese seem to have demonstrated the possibility of this approach. A Chinese physician in the 1950s noted that there were many childless marriages when crude cottonseed oil was used for cooking. That this was a male problem was easily demonstrated, because previously fertile men moving into the area became infertile.

Animal studies were completed in 1971, and these provided definitive proof of the efficacy and safety of the major constituent, gossypol. Clinical trials began in 1972 with men receiving a daily dose of 20 mg until their sperm counts dropped below an acceptable level. They then took a maintenance dose of 75–100 mg twice a month. Among the first 4000 men treated over periods ranging from six months to four years, the estimated efficacy of this regimen was 99.9 per cent, and there was complete recovery of acceptable sperm counts three months after the last dose of gossypol. Only time will tell whether this form of contraception is safe, effective, and acceptable to western men.

At the other end of the reproductive cycle, induction of labour has also exercised the intellects of the herbalists. In the Ebers papyrus we read that a woman should 'apply [peppermint] to her bare posterior' or alternatively the woman should take 'fennel, incense, garlic, sert-juice, fresh salt, wasp dung—make it into a ball and put it in the vagina'.

Of much greater therapeutic use was ergot, and this was first mentioned as an obstetric aid by the German physician Lonitzer in his *Kreuterbuch* published in 1582. European midwives accepted this suggestion with enthusiasm, and ergot was widely used to 'quicken labour'. The first scientific account of its use was given by the American physician John Stearns in 1808, though he admitted that his recipe for powdered ergot, or *pulvis parturens*, had originated from an immigrant German midwife.

It is interesting to compare the enthusiasm with which American physicians embraced this new drug with the more cautious approach taken by their European counterparts. The latter knew all about the dangers of ergotism, while the Americans had very little experience of this disease. As a consequence of this ignorance there was much over-prescribing and numerous maternal deaths and stillbirths resulted. In 1822 David Hosach of Columbia University advised caution and recommended its use solely as a means of stemming post-partum haemorrhage. This is nowadays the major obstetric use of the ergot alkaloids.

The isolation of the ergot alkaloids was studied at Burroughs Wellcome in 1903, and in 1905 Barger and Carr isolated a complex mixture of alkaloids that they called 'ergotaxine'. Later Stöll at Sandoz isolated pure ergotamine (in 1939), and Dudley, Moir, and co-workers at the National Institute for Medical Research in London obtained pure ergometrine. Kharasch, at the University of Chicago, also obtained ergometrine, though he called his compound ergonovine. This remains the best agent for the treatment of post-partum bleeding, and it causes a marked contraction of the uterine blood vessels.

Subsequent attempts by Stöll and Albert Hofmann to produce more potent compounds led to the discovery of LSD, which was discussed earlier. The structural relationship between LSD and ergometrine provided the basis for a highly imaginative, though illegal, drugs operation in the 1970s. A medically qualified member of the gang purchased large quantities of ergometrine, ostensibly for obstetric use, and a team of chemists then converted it into LSD. This lucrative business came to an abrupt end, thanks to the persistent efforts of the Thames Valley Police Force in an operation code-named 'Julie'.

While the various drugs and herbal remedies described so far directly affect the upper parts of the reproductive tract, the treatments given for venereal disease are mainly directed towards the lower parts of the urogenital tract. The causative organism of venereal syphilis, *Treponema pallidum*, only affects humans. There are three other distinct diseases caused by *Trepenoma* species: pinta, yaws, and endemic syphilis. Pinta and endemic or non-venereal syphilis are relatively mild conditions, and it is the other two diseases that have caused most of the suffering. In yaws the primary lesion usually appears on exposed parts of the body, while in venereal syphilis the first lesions appear on the genitalia. Subsequent spread to other parts of the body is most extensive in yaws, and bone damage is common. It is now clear that all four types of treponematoses were present in the Americas in pre-Columbian times, while in Europe only venereal and endemic syphilis were endemic. The strains of *Treponema* that cause pinta and yaws favour a hot, humid climate, while the other types grow best in a temperate environment.

Yaws was probably imported into Europe by the sailors returning from Columbus's voyages of discovery. They had probably contracted the disease in Haiti and what is now the Dominican Republic where the local Carib Indians were certainly afflicted. One of the chroniclers of Columbus's voyages, de Herrera, wrote in 1601 in his *General History* about events that he dated to 1503:

> *Due to their intercourse with the [Indian] women, they caught a disease common among the Indians, although unknown to the Castilians, that caused them great labour. There were pimples all over the body, accompanied by intense pains, contagious and without cure, which caused them to die cursing. Because of this, many of them returned to Castile, expecting to get better with the change of airs, but they spread the malady.*

There is no doubt about the location of the first epidemic, because this occurred during the invasion of Italy by the French army (which included some of Columbus's sailors) of Charles VIII. After the fall of Naples in 1495 there followed a period of unbridled licentiousness. Whether the French imported syphilis or contracted it from the Neapolitan whores is open to debate, but some of the latter were certainly Indians imported by the returning Spaniards, and were probably carriers of the disease. What is certain is that, when the French were finally driven from Italy, they took the disease with them and it was transmitted to the rest of the known world, claiming as many as ten million victims over the next fifteen years.

It was variously called the 'French disease', the 'Spanish disease', or the 'Great Pox', and those afflicted suffered initially with genital sores. There was then a rapid progression of the disease to involve the bones, with erosion of the palate and nose. At first the venereal aspect of the disease was not appreciated, and apart from cabbages the most often cited cause was blasphemy. Since sailors and soldiers swore most vociferously, it was quite natural that these should be the prime sufferers. Later the sin of fornication was implicated, and displays of passion during sexual intercourse were said to predispose the participants to contract the disease. Ambroise Paré (famous for his treatments for gunshot wounds) claimed that the disease was retribution from God: '. . . God's wrath, which allowed this malady to descend upon the human race, in order to curb its lasciviousness'. A more detailed account of the cause and effects was provided by Ulrich von Hutten, who caught the disease in his late teens. In particular, he identified the sexual link: 'There persist, within the private parts of women, lesions which remain remarkably virulent for a long time; they are particularly dangerous because they are less evident to the eye of the man who wishes to cohabit with women.'

Ultimately the South American Indians were blamed, probably to divert public attention from the cruel excesses of the *conquistadores*. The comments of the chronicler de Oviedo are typical: 'The first time this disease was seen, it was after Admiral Christopher Columbus discovered the Indies, and returned to these parts . . . those who were on the second voyage . . . brought this plague, and from them other people were contaminated.' He was fairly accurate in his comments about the mode of transmission: 'The disease is contracted most by intercourse of man with woman . . . few Christians who associate and have intercourse with Indian women have escaped from this danger.'

The name syphilis has a very interesting origin, since Syphilus was a major character and VD sufferer in the epic Latin poem (of 1530) called *Syphilis, sive Morbus Gallicus*, by Girolamo Fracastoro. Fracastoro is claimed to have been the greatest Latin poet since Virgil, but he was also a scientist and a philosopher. He was born in Verona in around 1483, and studied mathematics and medicine at the University of Padua, eventually becoming a lecturer in logic there in 1501. He wrote a number of books, and apart from the poem he is best known for his monumental work entitled *De Contagione*. In this he expounded his ideas of disease and its causes. In particular, he speculated that diseases were caused by 'particulas vero minimas et insensibles' (tiny invisible beings).

The poem contains a scientific account of the disease of syphilis, its causes, symptoms, and 'most important' the cures. Fracastoro advised that prevention was better than cure: 'keep away from Venus, and above all things avoid the soft pleasures of love-making—nothing is more harmful'; but for those afflicted a concoction of hops, fennel, parsley, fumitory, fern, maidenhair, spleenwort, squill, and hellebore could be applied to the sores. If this failed to effect a remission, more drastic measures were required: 'There are some who first of all heap together styrax, red mercuric sulphide and lead oxide, antimony and grains of incense, with whose bitter fumes they envelop the body entirely and destroy the deplorable disease.' Not surprisingly the patient suffered dreadfully: 'But the treatment is not only severe and fierce but also treacherous, since the breath chokes right in the throat and as it struggles free only with difficulty supports the ailing life.'

Mercurial ointments were the standard treatment right up until the advent of penicillin. They were popularized by Paracelsus in the sixteenth century, and their efficacy was demonstrated scientifically by Robert Koch in 1881 when he showed that mercuric chloride would kill anthrax spores growing in culture. The more soluble mercury salts, like the esters with benzoic acid and salicylic acid, were introduced in the late 1880s as a specific treatment for syphilis. Paul Erlich, the 'father' of medicinal chemistry, studied over 600 arsenic derivatives before discovering the highly potent arsenophenylglycine (arsphenamine, Salvarsan) in 1910. Between April and December 1910, some 65 000 vials of this drug were made available, free of charge, to physicians for the treatment of their patients, and this remained the drug of choice until penicillin became available.

A number of plants have received attention over the years, and extracts of the South American plants *Guaiacum sanctum* and *Guaiacum officinale*, lignum sanctum and lignum vitae respectively, were very popular in the sixteenth and seventeenth centuries. Gerard stated: 'The decoction of the barke or wood of *G. officinale* is of singular use in the cure of the French poxes, and it is the most ancient and powerful antidote that is yet known against that disease.' But the major contribution to prevention of the disease was made by a Dr Condon in the late eighteenth century. He fashioned what was colloquially known as the 'English frock coat' from the blind gut (caecum) of the lamb. This was washed, dried, and made pliable by treatment with almond oil, thus forming the first primitive condom. It will come as no surprise to learn that he was condemned by the clergy and praised by his customers. Then, as now, the device provided a fair degree of protection not only against impregnation but also against sexually transmitted diseases.

Finally, no self-respecting herbalist would have been without his recipes for love-potions and aphrodisiacs. Oberon asks for just such a potion in *Midsummer Night's Dream* (II, i):

> *Fetch me that flower; the herb I show'd thee once:*
> *The juice of it on sleeping eyelids laid*
> *Will make or man or woman madly dote*
> *Upon the next live creature that it sees.*

In humans the sex drive or libido in both men and women is under the control of a range of hormones including the hypothalamic hormone that stimulates the release of LH, prolactin, and testosterone. A number of plants figure on most lists of supposed aphrodisiacs, but yohimbine from the African tree *Corynanthe yohimbe* is probably the only one for which any evidence of efficacy can be given. Other, more doubtful, extracts include those from the vanilla bean, liquorice root, and ginseng. For at least the past 5000 years ginseng has been used by oriental men as a means of retaining or enhancing their virility. In controlled experiments it was shown to enhance stamina, and it probably acts as a general stimulant of metabolism.

A number of animal products are also noted for their legendary aphrodisiac properties. The most infamous of these are rhinoceros horn and dried blister beetles, so-called Spanish fly or cantharides from *Cantharis vesicatoria*. The former has no value, and the latter was always more likely to cause death rather than sexual arousal. Its reputation probably rests upon its ability to cause irritation of the urethra with resultant priapism, that is, prolonged stimulation of the erectile tissue in male or female genitalia.

In reality all of these potions and extracts are essentially useless, and the herbalists might have been more successful had they studied the effects of human secretions on members of the opposite sex. It is a well characterized phenomenon that most female mammals release odoriferous substances (sex pheromones) around the time of ovulation. These are sexually attractive (aphrodisiac) to the male, and mating takes place at the optimum time for successful propagation of the species. Human females secrete relatively large amounts of organic acids (e.g. acetic acid and butanoic acid) around the time of ovulation, and the odour of these could be best described as a mixture of vinegar and rancid butter. In addition, male sweat contains significant amounts of a breakdown product of testosterone that in concentrated form smells of urine. In trace amounts both types of chemicals have a musky odour which is not unattractive, and it is not impossible that these substances act as an aphrodisiac (released by the female) and dominance or submission factor (released by the male). In ancient times such chemical aids to successful sexual reproduction would clearly ensure propagation of the human species, which is more than can be said for the various herbal brews.

The heart and circulation

According to the Ebers papyrus the human heart functioned like a well rather than a pump, and the description of the heart and circulatory system was charming if somewhat confused: 'When the breath goes into the nose it makes its way to the heart and intestines, and the last-named vessels give to the body richly thereof . . . There are four vessels to his ears . . . breath-of-life goes in the right ear and breath-of-death into the left . . . There are two vessels to his testicles which convey the semen.' Their confusion over heart disease was more extreme: 'When the heart feels an aversion, behold it is the bitterness of the heart because of inflammation of the anus.' But their comprehension of heart failure was more accurate: 'When it is fate that he shall go up-on-high, behold it is the heart which determines that he shall go up-on-high.'

Despite attempts by Aristotle, Galen, and many others, only slow progress was made in understanding the mechanisms of the circulatory system. Galen believed that the arteries and veins comprised two separate systems, with a kind of tidal flow of blood to and from the heart. Venous blood was derived from digestion products in the liver and passed into the right side of the heart and thence to the lungs via the pulmonary artery. However, some venous blood leaked into the left side of the heart via 'communications', where it mixed with air from the lungs, thus generating a 'vital spirit', which was then transported around the body via the arteries. The major pumping role of the heart was clearly not recognized.

The Spaniard Michael Servetus (1509–1553) came closer to understanding the role of the heart. He was a theologian as well as a physician and he caused a great deal of displeasure among both Catholics and Protestants with his fierce Unitarian views. One of his religious texts, *The Restoration of Christianity*, contained an account of his ideas about the circulatory system. Like Galen he believed in the 'vital spirit', which had 'its source in the left ventricle of the heart, the lungs aiding most essentially in its production'. However, he denied the existence of a 'communication' in the heart, and suggested instead that 'the blood being transmitted from the pulmonary artery to the pulmonary vein, by a lengthened passage through the lungs, in the course of which it is elaborated and becomes a crimson colour'. In the lungs it 'mingles with the inspired air in this passage, and freed from fuliginous vapours' became a 'fit dwelling-place of the vital spirit'.

However, this useful scientific contribution was merely a side-issue compared with the heretical nature of the rest of his writing, and he was arrested in Geneva *en route* to Italy, tried for heresy, and burnt at the stake. It was then left to William Harvey (1578–1657) to give the first accurate account of the circulation of the blood.

Harvey was born in Kent and received his education at Cambridge and Padua, before taking a post as physician at St Bartholomew's Hospital in London. He was physician in turn to James I and Charles I, and announced his discoveries concerning the circulatory system in 1616. He completely demolished the theories of Galen concerning the 'communications' between the chambers of the heart, and showed that the blood was not consumed during its passage through the body. This last fact was very elegantly demonstrated when Harvey measured the volume of blood expelled by the heart over a period of several minutes, and showed that it far exceeded the total volume present in the body. Hence, it could not be replenished by the liver as Galen had suggested.

His book entitled *Exercitatio Anatomica de Motu Cordis et Sanguinis in Animalibus*, published in 1628, was written in Latin, but the translation that follows shows how perceptive he was:

First of all, the auricle contracts, and in the course of its contraction forces the blood ... into the ventricle, which being filled, the heart raises itself straightaway, makes all the fibres tense, contracts the ventricles and performs a beat, by which beat it immediately sends the blood supplied ... into the arteries. The right ventricle sends its charge into the lungs ... The left ventricle sends its charge into the aorta, and through this by the arteries to the body at large ... the one action of the heart is the transmission of the blood and its distribution, by means of the arteries, to the very extremities of the body.

This description is amazingly accurate, as can be seen from a consideration of Figs. 4.6 and 4.7. In an adult the heart is about the size of a man's fist and weighs between 180 and 400 g, depending upon stature and sex. It is a hollow organ made primarily from muscle (myocardial muscle), and it is divided into four chambers: the right and left atria and the right and left ventricles (see Fig. 4.6). Blood enters the heart via the atria and leaves via the ventricles (see Fig. 4.7). Oxygenated blood from the lungs enters the left atrium and passes into the left ventricle via the mitral valve, from where it is pumped through the aortic valve into the circulation via the aorta. The coronary arteries lead off the aorta, and supply blood to the walls of the heart. Deoxygenated blood returns to the right atrium via the large veins, the superior vena cava from the upper part of the body, and the inferior vena cava from the lower part of the body. This blood then passes into the right ventricle via the tricuspid valve and then via the pulmonic valve and the pulmonary artery to the lungs.

The coordination of the heart's pumping action (typically between seventy and eighty beats per minute at rest) is controlled by two groups of specialized muscle cells which are excitable and can conduct a nerve

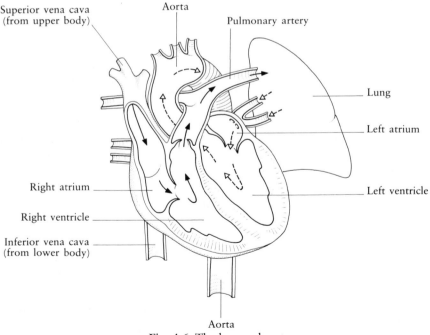

Fig. 4.6 The human heart.

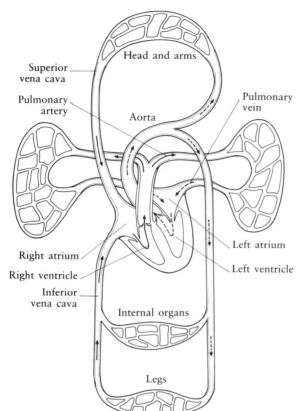

Superior vena cava

Pulmonary artery

Aorta

Head and arms

Pulmonary vein

Right atrium

Right ventricle

Inferior vena cava

Left atrium

Left ventricle

Internal organs

Legs

Fig. 4.7 Circulation of the blood.

impulse. These are known as the sinoatrial node and the atrioventricular node. All heart muscle is innervated and receives nerve signals via the autonomic system. When stimulated, the heart requires large volumes of oxygen to function efficiently, and this is why coronary artery disease is so debilitating and potentially dangerous.

During strenuous exercise the heart may need to increase its output tenfold, and the extra oxygen requirement is supplied by dilation of the coronary arteries. If this is not possible due to narrowing of the artery as a consequence of arteriosclerosis, the pain of angina is experienced. Arteriosclerosis is a major disease of developed countries where high fat diets are the norm, and it is caused by a build-up of fatty deposits in arterial walls. Stress, smoking, and excessive drinking all seem to exacerbate the condition, and in the heart the progressive deficiency in coronary blood supply is accompanied by the classic symptoms of heart disease: shortness of breath and fatigue on exercising, often accompanied by the pain of angina. A sudden occlusion of the coronary artery precipitates a heart attack (myocardial infarction), sometimes with associated disruption of the sinus rhythm. Death is most often due to the effects of these arrhythmias. The life-saving techniques of a sharp blow to the chest or the use of defibrillators owe their success to a restoration of the normal cardiac rhythm.

The long-term effects of heart disease also include various problems in other organs, most notably the kidneys; and the oedema (dropsy) that is probably caused by inefficient functioning of the kidneys is a common manifestation. Innumerable illustrations in medieval medical treatises show persons with fluid retention, especially with swellings of the arms and legs and a large paunch. Often the patient was bedridden, because the fluid filled the space around the lungs and made breathing difficult.

The ancient herbalists employed squill, or the sea onion, *Scilla maritima*, to treat the condition of dropsy. An old Syrian remedy employed 'wine of squills' for an 'evil condition of the liver and stomach, and for those who collect water'. Dioscorides claimed that 'the root . . . being smeared on with white wine upon boyes is thought to keep them impuberes'; but it also 'blindes ye belly and moves ye urine'. Gerard was also an enthusiastic prescriber: 'This roasted or baked onion is mixed with potions and other medicines which provoke urine, and open the stoppings of the liver and spleene . . . It is also given to those that have the dropsie, the yellow jaundice, and to such as are tormented with gripings of the belly.'

Other plant species that have been used through the ages include dogbane (*Apocynum cannabinum*) and various milkweeds (*Asclepias* species) which were much prized by the American Indians. All of these plants contain the so-called cardiac glycosides, which have already been mentioned as constituents of certain arrow poisons; but by far and away the most important source of these substances are the foxgloves *Digitalis purpurea* and *D. lanata*. In 1785 William Withering published his monograph *An Account of the Foxglove and some of its Medical Uses: with Practical Remarks on Dropsy, and other Diseases*. This was the first ever systematic evaluation of a drug and was a model of honest and thorough reporting, unrivalled until the clinical trials of the present century.

The origin of the word 'digitalis' is quite clear. It was first used by the German botanist Leonhardt Fuchs in 1542. In German the name for foxglove flowers was *Fingerhut*, or thimble, and hence the Latin word for finger, *digitus*, was adapted as a name for the plant species. The derivation

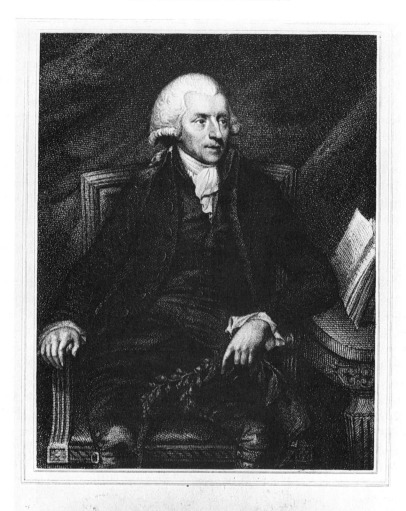

WILLIAM WITHERING M.D. F.R.S. &c. &c.

Drawn and Engraved by W. Bond, from an original picture

painted by C.F. Breda, in the possession of William Withering Esq.r F.L.S.

William Withering shown holding a foxglove, in an engraving by W. Bond (c. 1822). (Wellcome Institute Library, London.)

of the word 'foxglove' is much more obscure, but one plausible suggestion is that it is a corruption of 'folk's glove' (i.e. fairy's glove).

Extracts of the plant have been in use for many centuries, and Culpeper makes reference to its use for 'the king's evil' (i.e. scrofula, a form of TB). John Murray, professor of medicine in Hanover from 1769, was also enthusiastic about its medicinal value: 'A man with a scrophulous tumour of the right elbow, attended for three years with excruciating pains, and was nearly cured by four doses of the juice [*Digitalis purpurea*] taken once a month.'

The other major ailment for which it was prescribed was epilepsy. Culpeper claimed that 'a decoction of two handfulls thereof, with four ounces of polypody in ale has been found to cure divers of the falling sickness'. While John Parkinson claimed that 'after taking of the decoction . . . they that have been troubled with it [falling sickness] 26 years and have fallen once in a weeke . . . have not fallen once in 14 or 15 months'.

William Withering was certainly aware of these remedies, but until 1775 there is no evidence that he knew of its use for the treatment of dropsy. Withering was born in 1741 in Wellington, Shropshire, and not only was his father a successful apothecary but several other members of the family were either surgeons or physicians. With that pedigree it is not surprising that Withering was sent to study medicine (at Edinburgh University) and obtained his MD in 1766. After a brief spell in France, he returned to England and helped to set up the Stafford Infirmary, before moving to a practice in Birmingham in 1775. Throughout the rest of his life he treated both the rich and poor of Birmingham and pioneered the careful use of digitalis.

Withering completely dismissed the doctrine of signatures, which had held sway ever since the time of Galen, and stated on the first page of his book:

> As the more obvious and sensible properties of plants, such as colour, taste, and smell, have but little connection with the diseases they are adapted to cure; for their peculiar properties have no certain dependence upon external configuration . . . Their virtues must therefore be learnt, either from observing their effects upon insects and quadrupeds . . . or from the empirical usages and experience of the populace.

His interest in the use of the foxglove was aroused in 1775 by an enquiry concerning a secret remedy for dropsy that was prescribed by a Shropshire woman. The potion caused vomiting and purging, and contained the

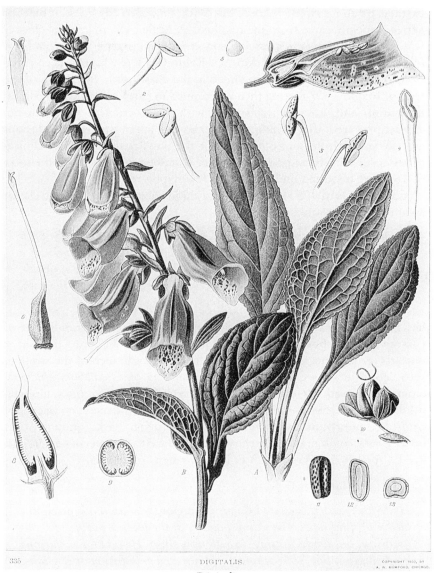

DIGITALIS.

Digitalis.

extracts of about twenty plants, but Withering correctly guessed that the active principle came from the foxglove. A further example of its efficacy was related to him soon after and concerned the Principal of Brazen Nose (now Brasenose) College, Oxford, Dr Ralph Cawley, who had been cured of a hydrops pectoris (dropsy affecting the chest) with an extract of the root of foxglove. Withering then determined to carry out a careful clinical evaluation and, after experimenting with a decoction of the plant (an extract prepared using boiling water), chose to administer either infusions (an extract with hot or cold water) or the powdered leaves. His clinical experiences with these preparations are described in his book in the form of 163 case histories, and they make fascinating reading.

Case IV (July 1775) concerned a middle-aged woman with classic symptoms of chronic heart failure:

> *I found her nearly in a state of suffocation; her pulse extremely weak and irregular, her breath very short and laborious, her countenance sunk, her arms of a leaden colour, clammy and cold . . . Her stomach, legs, and thighs were greatly swollen; her urine very small in quantity, not more than a spoonful at a time.*

She had been treated previously by Dr Erasmus Darwin, grandfather of Charles Darwin, but with no relief of her symptoms. Withering decided at once to try digitalis in admixture with nutmeg, and much of the swelling subsided. She subsequently received quantities of *Guaiacum officinale* (commonly used for the treatment of syphilis), myrrh, zinc sulphate, calomel (mercurous chloride), corrosive sublimate of mercury (mercuric chloride), potassium sulphate, rhubarb, Peruvian bark (quinine), and further doses of digitalis. Somehow she managed to survive all of this, and lived a further nine years with only minor signs of dropsy.

Case XX (January 1779):

> *Hydrops Pectoris; legs and thighs prodigiously anasarcous [accumulation of fluid under the skin especially in the legs] . . . urine in small quantity; pulse intermitting; breath very short. He had taken various medicines . . . but without relief . . . I directed an infusion of Digitalis, which made him very sick; acted powerfully as a diuretic, and removed all his symptoms.*

Case LXXI (May 1781):

> *Mr. S—, Aged 48. A strong man, who had lived intemperately. For some time past his breath had been very short, his legs swollen*

towards evening, and his urine small in quantity. Eight ounces of the Infus. Digitalis caused a considerable flow of urine; his complaints gradually vanished, and did not return.

Case LXXXI (October 1781):

Mr. B—, Aged 33. Had drank an immense quantity of mild ale, and was now become dropsical. He was a lusty man, of a pale complexion: his belly large, and his legs and thighs swollen to an enormous size. I directed the Infusion of Digitalis, which in ten days completely emptied him.

But not all the cases had such a successful conclusion, as for example with Case XIV (February 1778):

Mr. R— of K—. Had formerly suffered much from gout, and lived very intemperately. Jaundiced countenance; ascites [accumulation of fluid in the belly]; legs and thighs greatly swollen; appetite none; extremely weak; confined to his bed . . . I ordered him decoction of Digitalis, and a cordial; but he survived only a few days.

These many successes (and some failures) were achieved without any knowledge of the mode of action of digitalis. Withering never appreciated that the increased urinary flow and consequent relief of symptoms was due primarily to the increased contractility of heart muscle induced by the administration of digitalis. This ignorance should not detract from his major contributions to medicine, for not only did he carry out an exhaustive study of the effects of digitalis on his patients but he also stressed the importance of the careful choice of doses. This was much-needed advice, since most physicians at that time used large doses of cocktails of plant extracts.

After Withering's death in 1799 the use of digitalis declined. This was primarily because physicians tried to use it for every ailment imaginable, and their failure to effect cures of anything from bronchitis to mania led to a lack of confidence in the efficacy of digitalis. The physician Richard Bright published accounts of his clinical evaluations of digitalis in 1827 and correctly differentiated between dropsy due to kidney failure and that due to congestive cardiac failure, but his findings were largely ignored. A state of ignorance concerning the mode of action of digitalis existed right into the twentieth century.

In 1905 Sir James MacKenzie, the physician in charge of the heart wards at Mount Vernon Hospital in London, correctly recognized the condition of atrial fibrillation. He gave digitalis for this condition and noted that it enhanced the contractility of the heart (positive inotropic effect), but he believed that this was due to its slowing the heart rate. A better understanding of the effects of the drug was not possible until physicians had the use of an electrocardiograph. This was invented by Waller in 1887, with certain technological improvements made by Einthoven in 1903, and it allowed cardiologists to probe the different causes and sequelae of heart failure. It soon became clear that digitalis exerted a direct action on heart muscle and was beneficial in most types of heart failure, the notable exceptions being those caused by aortic valvular disease, e.g. aortic stenosis resulting from rheumatic fever.

Further advances had to await the isolation of the active constituents of digitalis. An active principle had been isolated in crude form from *D. purpurea* as early as 1841 by two Frenchmen, Homolle and Quevenne of the Hôpital de la Charité in Paris, and their efforts had been rewarded with a prize of 1000 francs from the Societé de Pharmacie. Other apparently different principles were isolated in the ensuing years, and there was much confusion until in 1928 Windaus and co-workers reported the actual structures of two major constituents, digitoxin and digitalin.

Two years later pure digoxin was isolated as a major component of *Digitalis lanata* by Sydney Smith of Burroughs Wellcome in Dartford, Kent. He showed that digoxin was more potent than anything from *Digitalis purpurea*, and Wellcome went on to market this natural product under the proprietary name Lanoxin. This is still widely used for the treatment of congestive heart failure. Initially Wellcome persuaded farmers in the Dartford area to grow *Digitalis lanata*, but because of the vagaries of the English climate most plants now come from warmer countries.

With the increasing clinical use of digoxin under careful conditions of dose and purity, it became apparent that its efficacy for different patients was very variable. In the first place, the digoxin tablets had to be carefully formulated such that there was efficient absorption of the drug, and as recently as the 1970s digoxin from different manufacturers had different efficacies.

The present view of its clinical utility can be summarized as follows: for patients with the heart arrhythmia called fast atrial fibrillation it is the drug of choice, but for patients with congestive cardiac failure (CCF) with no associated arrhythmia its use is more controversial. The mode of action of the cardiac glycosides like digoxin was explained in Chapter 1, but, to reiterate, it increases the contractility of heart muscle probably by increasing the intracellular availability of calcium ions. This results in increased cardiac output from the compromised heart after a heart attack.

Much more contentious is the use of digoxin for the long-term treatment of chronic CCF. Here many clinicians prefer to use diuretics rather than digoxin (to relieve the fluid retention), especially where the heart rhythm is normal. However, the long-term use of diuretics is not without hazard, and the advent of the synthetic vasodilators like captopril (Capoten) has provided a further option for treatment. These also help to lower the high blood pressure that is sometimes a consequence of the impaired kidney function in CCF. A further factor influencing the use of digoxin is its toxicity due to changes in the transport of sodium and potassium ions.

In a recent review in *Chemistry in Britain* celebrating the 200th anniversary of the publication of Withering's book, Aronson has neatly summarized the present position: 'In many centres the rates of intoxication and of therapeutic success associated with the use of digitalis are no better than those achieved by Withering at the end of the 18th century.' These reservations notwithstanding, William Withering's careful analysis of the use of a natural plant-derived drug still remains one of the milestones of drug discovery.

The high blood pressure referred to above is not only an occasional manifestation of heart disease, but also caused by malfunction as a consequence of kidney disease. A number of plant extracts have reputed antihypertensive activity, and the most often cited are those of the genus *Rauwolfia* and *Veratrum*. Extracts of *Rauwolfia* have been used for centuries in India. In Sanskrit the extract was known as *sarpagandha*, a legendary treatment for snakebite; and the Hindi name *chandra*, or 'moon', reflected its use as a tranquillizer for the treatment of lunacy. The major active constituent of *Rauwolfia* species is reserpine, and this acts by depleting catecholamine stores within the brain. As a result central sedative and tranquillizing effects are experienced, and in addition there is a relaxation of the heart and a lowering of blood pressure. In 1949, at the King Edward Hospital in Bombay, R. J. Vakil treated fifty patients suffering from high blood pressure with reserpine and obtained favourable results. His findings were confirmed by scientists at the Squibb Company in the USA, and reserpine was introduced into clinical use as an antihypertensive agent in 1953. It never realized its promise, but physicians noted that patients taking the drug became very relaxed, and it was subsequently developed as a tranquillizer. This facet will be discussed in the next section (on drugs affecting the nervous system).

One positive result of this failure was the experiments carried out by

Udenfriend at the National Heart Institute in Bethesda, Maryland. He knew that the synthetic drug methyldopa also induced a depletion of catecholamine stores, and this ultimately proved to be a very effective antihypertensive drug which was widely used before the introduction of more modern remedies such as the beta-blockers and captopril. As will be seen in the next section, the related drug L-dopa, also has interesting and useful actions upon the central nervous system.

The reduction of blood pressure, elimination of stress, and abstinence from smoking and heavy drinking are all possible ways of reducing the chances of a coronary. However, since the precipitating event is invariably a blockage in one of the blood vessels serving the heart, or the brain in the case of a stroke, there is considerable interest in drugs that act as anti-coagulants. There is no evidence that the ancients had any interest in this direction, but one of the commonly used drugs is certainly a structural analogue of a naturally occurring anticoagulant.

In the 1920s cattle in parts of North Dakota and Alberta suffered from a fatal haemorrhagic disease following the consumption of mouldy sweet clover. The causative factor was ultimately identified as dicoumarol, and although this natural product proved to be unsuitable for clinical use the totally synthetic analogue warfarin proved to be very effective. These compounds act by interfering with the body's blood-clotting mechanism, specifically at the stage involving vitamin K. Warfarin is perhaps better known as rat poison and it causes death through blood loss due to gastrointestinal haemorrhage.

Prevention is of course better than cure, and there is now very good evidence that garlic (and perhaps onion too) helps to prevent the formation of the atherosclerotic plaques that provide the nucleus for larger clots that cause the blockages in blood vessels. The ancient Egyptians and Babylonians consumed large quantities of garlic and onion, primarily for their supposed magical properties. The seafaring Vikings and Phoenicians also avoided scurvy by taking quantities of garlic (and its constituent vitamin C) on their sea voyages. The Jews were also fond of garlic, but it is said that the recommendation in the Talmud to 'eat garlic on Friday on account of its salutary action' referred to its supposed aphrodisiac properties. In contrast, the Muslims have a disdain for the strong smell of garlic, though they were not above using it to ward off the 'evil eye'. In fact it was common practice in many countries to wear amulets made from garlic to ward off vampires and other evil things.

For clinical use Dioscorides recommended garlic for snake bite, rabid-dog bite, bloodshot eyes, baldness, eczema, herpes, leprosy, scurvy, toothache, and dropsy, while Pliny in his *Natural History* extolled its virtues for the same conditions and also as an antidote against henbane and aconite poisoning, asthma, haemorrhoids, catarrh, convulsions, and ruptures. Culpeper reported similar usage:

> *It provokes urine, and women's courses, helps the biting of mad dogs and other venomous creatures, kills worms in children, cuts and voids tough phlegm, purges the head, helps the lethargy, is a good preservative against, and a remedy for any plague, sore, or foul ulcers; takes away spots and blemishes in the skin, eases pains in the ears. . .*

Only recently its probable prophylactic efficacy against arteriosclerosis has been discovered. A number of garlic constituents have been identified in recent years, and two of these, ajoene and methylallyl trisulphide, have marked activity as inhibitors of blood platelet aggregation. Since this kind of aggregation or clumping is a major contribution to clot formation, it is hardly surprising that in countries where the consumption of garlic is high, the death rate from coronaries is relatively low. For example, the UK has a very high incidence of heart attack (1800 per 100 000 of the male population aged 35–75 per year), while in France the comparable figure is 150 per 100 000 (1987 figures from the British Heart Foundation). Other factors must of course be taken into consideration, but the prophylactic effect of garlic must certainly be taken seriously. When Culpeper stated that 'it is a remedy for all diseases and hurts', his overstatement was perhaps nearer the truth than might be imagined.

Drugs affecting the central nervous system
Analgesics

> Not poppy, nor mandragora,
> Nor all the drowsy syrups of the world,
> Shall ever medicine thee to that sweet sleep
> Which thou ow'dst yesterday.
>
> Othello, *III, iii*

The ancients were well aware of the sleep-inducing properties of mandrake and opium, and although the former was also much used to relieve pain, it is the opium poppy that provides the most famous (and infamous) analgesic of all—morphine. The Sumerians certainly used opium as early as 4000 BC. In the Ebers papyrus it appears as part of a remedy for a colicky child:

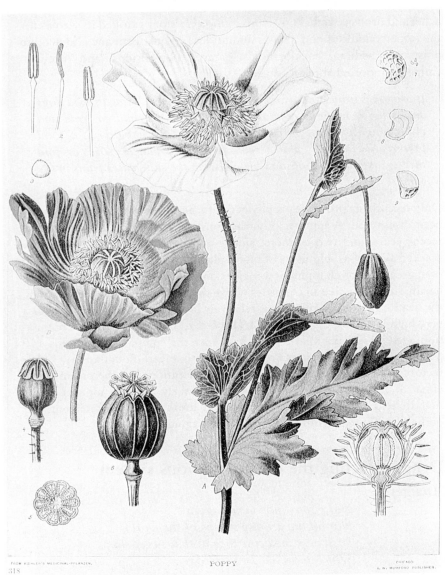

FROM KOHLER'S MEDICINAL-PFLANZEN.
318
POPPY
CHICAGO.
A. W. MUMFORD, PUBLISHER.

The opium poppy (*Papaver somniferum*).

'pods of the poppy plant, fly dirt which is on the wall'. In Greek mythology the opium poppy was dedicated to Thanatos (god of death), Hypnos (god of sleep), and Morpheus (god of dreams), and Homer in the *Odyssey* has Helen prepare a drugged wine 'that banishes all care, sorrow, and ill humour'. The actual collection of crude opium was first described by Dioscorides:

> *But it behoves them that make opium . . . to scarify about the asterisk [the small star on the head of the seed capsule] with a knife . . . and from the sides of the head make straight incisions in the outside, and to wipe off the tear that comes out with the finger into a spoon, and again to return not long after, for there is found another [tear] thickened, and also on the day after.*

This method of collection is still used, and opium is defined as the dried, milky exudate that emerges if unripe seed capsules of *Papaver somniferum* are scored. This brown, gummy mass contains about 25 per cent by weight of opium alkaloids, of which morphine (up to 17 per cent by weight) and codeine (up to 4 per cent) are the most important.

Galen prescribed opium for, among other conditions, chronic headache, vertigo, epilepsy, asthma, colic, fevers, dropsies, leprosies, melancholy, and 'troubles to which women are subject'. This wide spectrum of activities endeared it to physicians and patients alike, and its fame and use spread with the successive waves of Arabian invaders and traders. In the century following the death of Mohammed in AD 632, the Arab empire grew until it extended from Spain in the west to India in the east. Opium was thus introduced into Persia, India, and what is now Malaysia during the eighth century, and during the Middle Ages into China. Soon it was under cultivation in all of these countries, and was primarily used as a sleeping draught and treatment for diarrhoea.

Its use as an analgesic was popularized by Paracelsus in the sixteenth century when he introduced various preparations of opium under the name 'laudanum' (from the Latin *laudare*, to praise). Thomas Sydenham (famous for his extracts of cinchona bark, i.e. quinine) is credited with the introduction of opium into Britain, but it was his pupil, Thomas Dover, who invented the much-valued Dover's powder. Dover was an interesting character, a one-time pirate and rescuer of Alexander Selkirk (Defoe's model for Robinson Crusoe), who then took up medicine. His powder contained opium, liquorice, saltpetre, and ipecacuanha, with the latter ingredient acting rather conveniently as an emetic should the prescribed dose be exceeded. Another popular remedy was Godfrey's cordial, which contained opium, molasses, and sassafras, and this was much used as a teething aid, for rheumatic pains, and for diarrhoea.

Until the early seventeenth century, the Chinese had mainly used opium as an ingredient in cakes for special occasions and as a medicine, but it was the arrival of tobacco that precipitated the sudden interest in opium smoking. After its discovery in the fifteenth century, tobacco-smoking became very popular among sailors, and these introduced the habit into China, India, Japan, and Siam (Thailand). In China smoking became so widespread that the Emperor Tsung Chen prohibited the use of tobacco in 1644, with the result that the population turned to opium instead. By the end of the century about one-quarter of the population were using the drug. The local crop was insufficient to supply the needs of this vast clientele, and the British East India Company began a lucrative trade that sought to satisfy this need. By the 1830s the Company was supplying £1 000 000 worth of opium per annum, which represented about one-sixth of the total annual Indian revenue of the Company. Most of this opium was smuggled into China via the port of Canton by British and American merchants, and eventually in 1839 the Chinese authorities took steps to stem this flow of illicit opium.

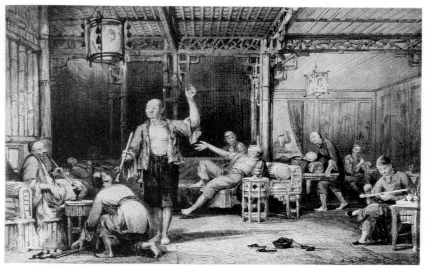

A nineteenth century Chinese opium den. (Wellcome Institute Library, London.)

The Chinese government appointed a commissioner named Lin Tse-Hsu to undertake this task, and after several false starts he succeeded in seizing and destroying 1000 tons of opium in March of 1839. A minor riot ensued, and he then closed the port of Canton to the British to prevent further importation. Tempers frayed, shots were fired, and the first Opium War began in November 1839. This lasted until 1842, during which time a force of 10 000 British troops and sailors captured or blockaded several ports, and eventually the Chinese were forced to capitulate. At the subsequent peace conference in Nanking, the Chinese ceded Hong Kong to the British in perpetuity (though it will now be restored to them in 1997), and were forced to concede greater trading rights and £21 000 000 in reparations. The import of opium was renewed with even greater vigour.

Over the succeeding years the morality of this trade was questioned from time to time. In 1893 a motion in the British parliament that the 'opium trade was morally indefensible' was defeated by a large majority and a Royal Commission produced a lengthy report, but no action was taken. At least part of the problem was the high degree of ignorance and prejudice that existed, as evidenced by the following statement from an 1882 report entitled 'The Opium Question Solved': 'If Indian opium was stopped at once it would be a very frightful calamity indeed. I should say that one-third of the adult population [of China] would die for want of opium.' Finally, in 1908, Britain resolved to reduce exports of Indian opium to China, but it was the introduction of opium into the USA, Australia, and South America by Chinese immigrants that finally persuaded the various governments that action had to be taken to curb the use of the narcotic.

The International Opium Commission was inaugurated in 1909, and by 1914 thirty-four nations had agreed to curb opium production and importation. World War I then intervened, and at the Commission's next meeting in 1924 the number of countries that had agreed to some form of control had risen to sixty-two. Finally, the newly formed League of Nations took over the task of controlling opium and other narcotics, and among other resolutions declared that all signatory countries should pass 'effective laws or regulations to limit exclusively to medical and scientific purposes the manufacture, import, sale, distribution, export, and use of all narcotic drugs'. These were admirable goals, but the poor farmers of India, Pakistan, Afghanistan, Turkey, Iran, and the so-called 'Golden Triangle', where the borders of Burma, Thailand, and Laos converge, were little affected by such noble sentiments. To them the production of illicit opium was far more worthwhile than subsistence farming. The illicit trade continued to flourish and still does.

One of the reasons for the popularity of opium, and more recently heroin, has been its association with artists. Writers like Thomas de Quincey, Edgar Allan Poe, and Samuel Taylor Coleridge must shoulder at least some of the blame for the spread of opiate use in Europe and America. De Quincey is said to have first tried laudanum in 1804 to relieve the pains of toothache and rheumatism. His enthusiasm for the drug knew no bounds:

> *That my pains had vanished was now a trifle in my eyes; this negative effect was swallowed up in the immensity of these positive effects which had opened before me, in the abyss of divine enjoyment thus suddenly revealed.*

Later he described his love affair with opium in more poetic terms:

> *O just, subtle and all-conquering opium! ... O just and righteous opium! that to the chancery of dreams summonest, for the triumphs of despairing innocence, false witnesses ... and, 'from the anarchy of dreaming sleep', callest into sunny light the faces of long buried beauties ... and thou hast the keys of Paradise, O just, subtle and mighty opium!*

His recollections of his years with opium were subsequently recorded in his most famous work entitled *Confessions of an English Opium Eater* published in 1821.

It is certain that Coleridge was aware of the 'joys of opium', and he was consuming around four pints of laudanum a week at the time of his greatest creativity. If one reads *The Rime of the Ancient Mariner*, it is easy to imagine that opium played some part in the creation of this unusual poem:

> *Yea, slimy things did crawl with legs*
> *Upon the slimy sea.*
> *About, about, in reel and rout*
> *The death-fires danced at night;*
> *The water, like a witch's oils,*
> *Burnt green, and blue and white.*

Chemical investigations of opium began in the nineteenth century, and in 1804 Armand Séquin first isolated the major constituent, which he christened 'morphine' after the Greek god of dreams. A year later Friedrich

Wilhelm Serturner, who had been trained as an apothecary, also isolated morphine and established its narcotic potency on a dog. Although he published his results, they were ignored until a further publication appeared in 1917 in the prestigious *Annales de Chimie*. This told of his experiences after overdosing with 100 mg of morphine.

With the invention of the hypodermic syringe in 1853, the means were available for the effective relief of pain, and morphine was widely used for this purpose during the American Civil War and the Franco-Prussian War. In 1874, Alder Wright of St Mary's Hospital Medical School prepared an analogue of morphine, diacetylmorphine (diamorphine), and this was marketed by the German company Bayer in 1898. It was hailed as a 'heroic' drug, hence the name heroin, and was widely used especially in cough remedies. Its highly addictive nature was not appreciated until later, by which time it had gained world-wide popularity, and governments then had to rapidly introduce new legislation governing the use of dangerous drugs.

The chemical structure of morphine was first proposed in 1923 by John Gulland and Robert Robinson, but the first chemical synthesis was not achieved until 1952 by Gates and Tschudi, and an X-ray crystallographic study was not completed until 1968, 164 years after the original isolation by Séquin. Over the years numerous structural analogues of morphine have been prepared by the pharmaceutical industry in an attempt to produce a potent analgesic that lacks the addictive potential of morphine and heroin. In the early years these investigations had to be carried out without any knowledge of the mode of action of morphine, and most of the analogues were simpler chemical structures like levorphanol, dextro-methorphan, and pethidine (known as meperidine in the USA). This last drug has proved to be particularly effective for the relief of pain associated with childbirth, and an added bonus is that it does not depress the baby's respiration as much as morphine. A comparison of the structures of pethidine and morphine is shown in Fig. 4.8.

The mode of action of the opiates is still only partially understood, but it is now possible at least to identify the sites at which they exert their analgesic and euphoriant effects. Morphine and the other opiates bind to receptors in the brain and elsewhere. The identification of these opioid receptors was facilitated by the use of two kinds of opiate analogue: the synthetic opiate antagonists like naloxone, and opiates labelled with tritium, a radioactive isotope of hydrogen.

The opiate antagonists arose as part of the programme directed to-wards the design of novel opiates which lacked addictive potential while

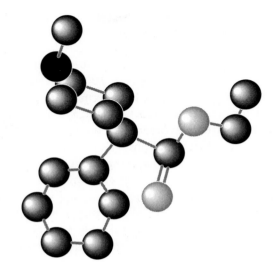

Pethidine

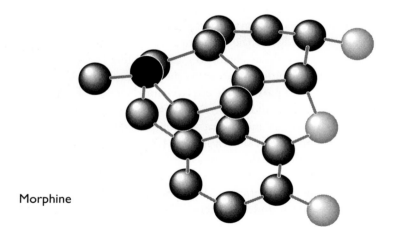

Morphine

Fig. 4.8 Comparison of the structures of pethidine and morphine.

retaining analgesic potency. They antagonize the effects of morphine and heroin by displacing them from their receptors, but once bound they do not elicit the typical euphoriant response. This is how naloxone functions when given to reverse the effects of a heroin overdose.

The tritiated analogues have one or more tritium atoms in place of hydrogen atoms. These atoms are radioactive and the molecules thus emit β-particles, the number of which can be detected. Using these two types of analogues, Pert and Snyder were able to show in 1973 that morphine, naloxone, and other opiates did indeed bind to discrete receptors in brain tissue and in the gastrointestinal tract. The actual location of the receptors was more difficult to determine, but ultimately in 1975 Pert, Snyder, and Kuhar—all of the Johns Hopkins University Medical School in Baltimore— achieved this goal. They found the highest concentrations of receptors in those areas of the brain known to be involved in pain perception, the substantia gelatinosa and the thalamus (Fig. 4.9). In addition there was a dense aggregation of receptors in an area close to the cerebral cortex known as the limbic region. This was particularly interesting, because cells in this area were known to be involved in the control of emotional behaviour. The limbic region also has connections to the hypothalamus, which as we have seen has a major role in the control of hormone release,

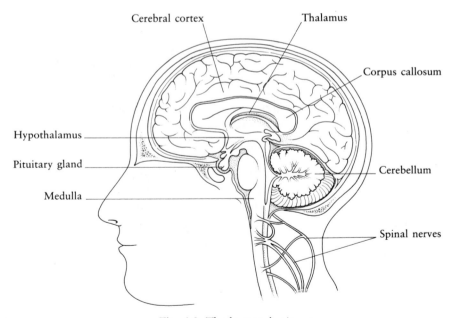

Fig. 4.9 The human brain.

thus explaining how the opiates might have a wider influence over mood. Other peripheral receptors (e.g. in the gut) are obviously associated with the gastrointestinal calmative effect of morphine.

The mechanism of addiction is less clear, but it is not simply due to changes in the number of receptors or in their biochemical properties. The only certain fact is that habitual users of opiates require increasing quantities of the drugs to satisfy the craving and suffer severe withdrawal symptoms upon removal of the drug. Coleridge's poem 'Dejection' could well have been written while he was suffering such withdrawal. Possibly the most suggestive lines are:

> *Hence, viper thoughts, that coil around my mind,*
> *Reality's dark dream!*
> *I turn from you, and listen to the wind,*
> *Which long has rav'd unnotic'd. What a scream*
> *Of agony by torture lengthen'd out*
> *That lute sent forth!*

All of this information concerning receptors immediately posed one fundamental question: why does the brain have receptors for a plant alkaloid? The obvious explanation was that the brain produces its own endogenous opiate-like substance, and several research groups began a search for these hypothetical substances. The first to conclusively demonstrate their existence were Hughes and Kosterlitz of Aberdeen University in 1975. They isolated two pentapeptides (five amino acids joined together in a defined sequence) which bound to opioid receptors and elicited analgesic activity. They christened these 'enkephalins' (from the Greek *kephalē*, head), though the preferred American name was 'endorphins' and this name now includes the enkephalins and other more recently discovered peptides with opiate activity. A comparison of the structures of an enkephalin and morphine is shown in Fig. 4.10.

The enkephalins were subsequently shown to be true neurotransmitters that bind to opioid receptors at dopaminergic and cholinergic centres in both the brain and the gut. However, the situation has become more complex of late with the discovery that there are at least three types of opioid receptor, so-called μ, κ, and δ receptors. The μ receptor is the primary point at which morphine binds and exerts its biological effects, and it appears to be responsible for analgesia, euphoria, addiction, and respiratory depression. The κ receptor mediates analgesia and sedation, while the δ receptor is the main point of binding for the enkephalins, and presumably mediates their analgesic effect, though it also appears to be

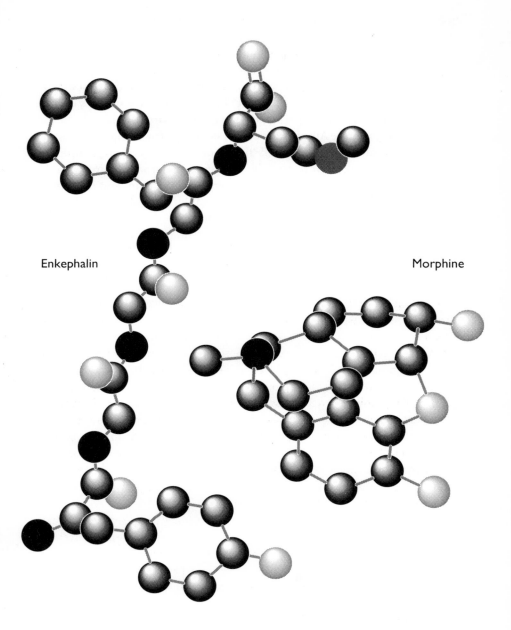

Enkephalin

Morphine

Fig. 4.10 Comparison of the structures of an enkephalin and morphine.

involved with psychotomimetic effects. At the μ receptor the binding of an agonist initiates the opening of potassium ion channels on the neurons, with resultant hyperpolarization and inhibition of neurotransmission. Binding of an agonist at the δ receptor causes inhibition of adenyl cyclase, with a consequent reduction in the production of the secondary messenger cyclic AMP. Finally, binding of an agonist at a κ receptor induces closure of calcium channels, with a resultant lowering of intracellular concentrations of calcium ions. All of these events (summarized in Fig. 4.11) either reduce the frequency of nerve-cell 'firing' or precipitate changes in intracellular biochemistry that restrict the synthesis of neurotransmitters. In the brain this results in a diminution in the perception of pain, and this is why the opioid-like drugs (opiates) are so valuable as analgesics. The true opioids also induce euphoria and sedation, and their most dangerous adverse effect, apart from their addictive potential, is a depression of the respiratory centre of the brain.

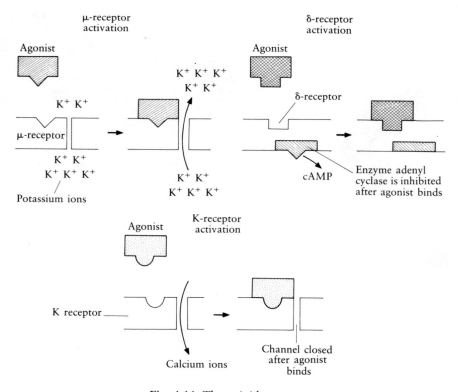

Fig. 4.11 The opioid receptors.

With this greater understanding of receptor type and location has come the ability to design novel opiates with specific biological activity. Thus, buprenorphine has a very high affinity for all three types of receptor, but appears to be an agonist at the κ and δ receptors, while having potent antagonist activity at μ receptors. This makes it an effective analgesic essentially devoid of addictive potential. Another interesting development is the design of novel bis-opiate molecules by Portoghese and co-workers. These comprise two opiate-like structures held in such a way that they can interact with two neighbouring receptors at the same time. This should allow the production of molecules that position an antagonist at a μ site and an agonist at a κ site, again with resultant analgesia without addiction.

Gerard very succinctly summarized the two extreme actions of opium: '... taken either inwardly, or outwardly applied to the heade, provokes sleepe. Opium somewhat too plentifully taken doth also bring death.' Modern pharmacy owes a lot to this plant drug, but it is no longer necessary to accept both its positive and negative features. In the forseeable future, there is the realistic probability of rationally designed non-addictive analgesic drugs.

At the 'street' level a different kind of drug design has also been pursued, often with devastating results. As well as the synthesis of heroin, which is a multi-billion pound business, and Ectasy, two other designer drugs have achieved notoriety. One of these, phencyclidine (PCP) was originally introduced as a clinically useful general anaesthetic in the 1950s. However, a proportion of patients suffered a period of disorientation on emerging from their anaesthesia, and many appeared to experience a type of schizophrenia. The drug was 'rediscovered' in the 1970s, and its street sobriquets Angel Dust and DOA (dead on arrival) indicate its effects and possible consequences. In modest doses the drug causes hallucinations, but when taken in overdoses acute schizophrenia and coma often result. It has been suggested that it exerts its effects through binding to a fourth type of opioid receptor (σ), but it also reduces the release of the neurotransmitter glutamic acid in the brain.

The other designer drug has even more insidious effects. This was sold in northern California in the early 1980s and was known as MPTP (1-methyl-4-phenyl-4-(1,2,3,6-tetrahydropyridine)), or 'synthetic heroin'. It produced very alarming symptoms in those taking it intravenously. These included not only hallucinations but also near total immobility and an inability to talk intelligibly. These symptoms were broadly similar to those exhibited by patients with advanced types of Parkinson's disease. It is probable that the drug users suffered a destruction of brain cells in the region of the brain (substantia nigra) known to be most affected in Parkinson's disease. An understanding of the actual mode of action of MPTP is thus of interest in order to understand the aetiology of this disease.

Tranquillizers and other drugs

While the treatment of pain is now almost wholly scientific, the treatment of mental illness is of necessity much more tentative, given the general state of ignorance that exists regarding the causes of such illness. A lot of the treatment still relies on the use of tranquillizers, and one natural plant drug, reserpine, has proved of great value both for therapy and as an aid to understanding neurological disorders. The drug is derived from the root of the plant *Rauwolfia serpentina*, which is a native of the Indian subcontinent, and has been used for centuries to treat a whole range of ailments. The plant was first imported into Europe by the German botanist Leonhard Rauwolf—hence the name. The primary folk use for the extract was as a means of attaining states of introspection and meditation, and Indian holy men, including Mahatma Ghandi, were habitual users of the drug.

In 1952, Emil Schlitter isolated reserpine and demonstrated its tranquillizing activity. In clinical use it showed marked antihypertensive activity, and ultimately this property was valued rather than its potential as a tranquillizer. However, as millions of patients with high blood pressure took the drug, a large number began to exhibit symptoms of depression, and these were severe enough to cause a number of suicides. At about the same time it became possible to estimate concentrations of brain amines, and it was demonstrated that reserpine caused a depletion of the central brain amines serotonin, dopamine, and noradrenalin. This was effected by an inhibition of re-uptake of the amines into the neurons which normally released them.

This feature of the drug's activity was, for a while, used in the treatment of schizophrenia (from the Greek *skhizō*, split, and *phrēn*, mind), a disease in which there is little connection between thoughts and actions. Those afflicted are usually introverted and suffer from strange delusions. Elevated concentrations of dopamine are believed to be a major cause of the condition. One adverse effect of reserpine use was a condition resembling Parkinson's disease, and patients suffered tremors, muscular rigidity, and weakness. This was historically very important, since it presaged the observation that dopamine was grossly depleted in people suffering from Parkinson's disease. Before 1957 dopamine had been thought to be merely a precursor of noradrenalin and adrenalin, but these findings suggested that it must have a neurotransmitter role of its own. This led in 1967 to the introduction of L-dopa (L-dihydroxyphenylalanine) as an effective treatment for Parkinson's disease. Dopamine itself cannot be used, since it does not cross the blood/brain barrier. This is a membranous type of structure that effectively excludes charged molecules (those bearing ionic charges) from the brain, and those drugs that do gain entry usually succeed via diffusion from one aqueous medium (blood) to another aqueous medium (cerebrospinal fluid). L-dopa will cross this barrier, and since it is the immediate precursor to dopamine it provides a means of increasing local concentrations of dopamine.

The other increasingly common form of senile brain dysfunction is Alzheimer's disease, and this appears to be associated with a deficiency of acetylcholine in the central nervous system. The concentrations can be as low as 30 per cent of normal, and at present there is no simple precursor molecule (like L-dopa) that can be administered to patients. Treatment of this disease promises to be one of the challenges of the twenty-first century, since around 20 per cent of the population will then be over 65 years old.

Migraine is another condition that has afflicted mankind since the dawn of time, and this may also be responsive to natural drug therapy. The early monastic apothecaries used feverfew (*Tanacetum parthenium*) as a treatment for both migraine and arthritis, and Gerard, as usual, provided a near poetic description of its use: 'very good for them that are giddie in the head, or which have the turning called Vertigo, that is, a swimming and turning in the head'.

Until recently there was no real evidence that extracts of the plant were effective. However, in 1985, a study at the London Migraine Clinic provided some indication that feverfew had prophylactic efficacy, though the findings were complicated by the irregular constitution of the plants. The major active constituents are said to be parthenolide and related structures, and these are known to vary widely in composition between plants and with the seasons.

The proposed mode of action of these compounds involves inhibition of release of serotonin from blood platelets within the brain, and this could also explain the claimed utility of the extract in the treatment of arthritis and psoriasis. It is certainly true that there are changes in cerebral blood flow during a migraine attack, and other clinically useful drugs like ergotamine may be effective because they cause constriction of blood vessels. As to the importance of serotonin in the aetiology of the condition, it is unclear whether a deficit or excess of the neurotransmitter is involved. The ergot alkalkoid derivative methysergide is an effective prophylactic agent, and may function (in small doses) as a serotonin (5-hydroxytryptamine) antagonist. Similarly, the new Glaxo drug, Sumatriptan, which is a structural analogue of 5-hydroxytryptamine, also has serotonin-like activity.

The actual mode of action of all of these drugs is still unresolved, and the efficacy and safety of feverfew are not proven. It would be a shame if its folkloric use proved to be totally without foundation, though we should still be left with Culpeper's claim that 'it is an especial remedy against opium taken too liberally'.

Anti-asthma drugs

Much of the herbology concerning the treatment of afflictions of the lungs and upper respiratory tract was directed towards remedies for coughs and colds. Culpeper recommended rosemary (*Rosmarinus officinalis*): 'The dried leaves shred small, and taken in a pipe, as tobacco is taken, helps those that have any cough, phthisic, or consumption.' A more alcoholic recipe appeared in *Bancke's Herbal*: 'If you have a cough drink the water of the leaves [of rosemary] boyled in white wine, and ye shall be whole.'

Unfortunately, most infections of the upper respiratory tract are due to viruses, so the cough and cold remedies would have been palliative at best. A cure for the common cold still eludes us, and there is unlikely ever to be a single treatment, since there are dozens of viral serotypes involved. One controversial treatment involves the use of multigram quantities of vitamin C. This was pioneered by Linus Pauling, twice winner of the Nobel prize (for chemistry in 1954 and peace in 1963). He is not alone in his beliefs, and we all know people who swear by their hot lemon drinks or large doses of vitamin C tablets. However, although the vitamin may well be effective during the recovery phase of a cold, its clinical efficacy as a preventive agent has not been established.

Herbal remedies made a much more effective contribution to the treatment of asthma, and two major drugs have arisen more or less directly from folk medicine. Asthma is caused by a generalized bronchoconstriction (narrowing of the airways), usually associated with inflammation and excessive secretion of mucus. The prevalence of asthma in the UK is around 5 per cent and rising, and the lungs of all sufferers are hyperresponsive to a variety of stimuli. These may include not only typical allergens, like ragweed pollen, house dust, and animal fur, but also smoke, cold air, and even exercise. Some asthmatics respond to all of these stimuli.

Herbal remedies have relied on three tried and tested strategies: the use of various *Ephedra* species, especially *E. equisetina* and *E. sinaica*; the use of plants containing xanthines like caffeine and theophylline; and plants that contain tropane alkaloids. For example, the American Indians smoked the leaves of *Lobelia inflata*, while in India the whole of *Lobelia nicotianaefolia* was used for the treatment of both bronchitis and asthma. Both of these plants contain the tropane alkaloid lobeline. The smoking of jimsonweed (*Datura stramonium*) has already been mentioned, and a number of tropane alkaloids related in structure to atropine (e.g. ipratropium) have been used for inhalation by asthmatics. The Chinese have been using Ma Huang, an extract from the two *Ephedra* species, for at least the last 5000 years, but the active constituent, ephedrine, was not isolated until 1887. At about the same time the work on the sympathomimetic amines began, and this was to lead eventually to the discovery of salbutamol and related anti-asthmatic drugs. A comparison of the structures of adrenalin, ephedrine, and salbutamol is shown in Fig. 4.12.

In 1897 the American physician Jacob Abel isolated what he believed to be a rejuvenating factor from sheep adrenal (epinephric) glands, and christened it epinephrine. A few years later, a more efficient extraction method was devised, and the pharmaceutical company Parke Davis marketed epinephrine under the name adrenalin. During the early years of the twentieth century, Friedrich Stölz, head of chemical research at Hoechst Dyeworks in Germany, supervised the synthesis of a number of analogues of adrenalin, one of which was noradrenalin. It was not until 1946 that the key role of noradrenalin as a neurotransmitter was established by Ulv von Euler, but in the meantime it was soon realized that many of these analogues of adrenalin had a potent effect on the sympathetic nervous system. They were thus christened the 'sympathomimetics', but their potential clinical utility was not appreciated until much later.

In 1923 at the Peking Union Medical College, Ku Kuei Chen was investigating the medicinal properties of Ma Huang prepared from *Ephedra sinaica* and managed to obtain pure ephedrine. Experiments with dogs showed that the compound produced a sustained rise in blood pressure and heart rate after intravenous injection, and these effects were similar to those elicited by adrenalin. It was subsequently licensed for clinical use in 1926, and became the first orally active bronchodilator for use by asthmatics.

Other related structures were prepared, and the amphetamines proved to be of particular pharmacological interest. The Benzedrine (amphetamine) inhaler was introduced to ease nasal congestion, and both Benzedrine and Methedrine (methylamphetamine) were widely used during World War II as central nervous system stimulants. After the war they were widely available both legally and illegally, and serious abuse resulted. These effects on the central nervous system were not desirable for an anti-asthma

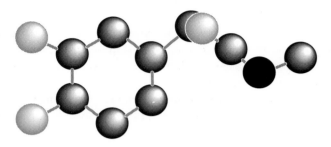

Adrenaline

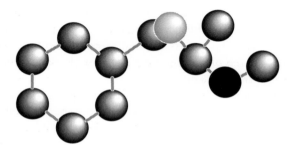

Ephedrine

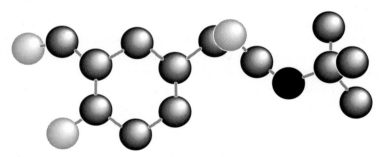

Salbutamol
(Ventolin)

Fig. 4.12 Comparison of the structures of adrenaline, ephedrine, and salbutamol.

drug, and further permutations in structure were required before the appropriate pharmacological profile was achieved.

By combining the ring structure of adrenalin or ephedrine with a hybrid adrenalin/amphetamine side-chain, the drug isoprenaline (known as isoproterenol in the USA) was obtained. This was introduced as a bronchodilator in 1951 and proved highly popular, especially among young asthma sufferers. Unfortunately, although it had little effect on blood pressure, it had marked cardiac stimulant properties, and many teenagers unknowingly took large overdoses from their inhalers. In the UK alone, 3000 deaths from resultant cardiac arrest were recorded before the drug was withdrawn.

Other structural modifications were needed in order to provide drugs with long-lasting bronchodilator activity without the associated cardiac adverse effects. The two most successful products of this drug design were salbutamol (Ventolin, Glaxo), and terbutaline (Bricanyl, Astra), and these are currently the most widely used anti-asthma drugs. The selectivity of these drugs is due to their specific interaction with certain adrenalin receptors (β_2-adrenoceptors) in the lungs. Unlike adrenalin, which interacts with β-adrenoceptors in the lungs and the heart (β_2 and β_1 receptors respectively), the newer drugs are essentially devoid of actions at the β_1 receptors. Despite the subtle engineering of their chemical structures to improve efficacy, their lineage from Ma Huang and the Chinese herbs is still plain to see.

These drugs, though invaluable, only treat the symptoms of asthma, and it is better to have preventive agents. As we saw in the section on inflammation, an asthmatic attack is often precipitated by the binding of allergens to antibodies on the surface of mast cells. This binding initiates the opening of calcium channels and the in-rush of calcium ions triggers various enzymatic reaction within the mast cells. These in turn lead to the synthesis and subsequent release of histamine, prostaglandins, leukotrienes, and other factors that cause bronchoconstriction or inflammation. The antihistamines and the bronchodilators diminish the effects of these mediators, but do nothing to prevent their synthesis or release. The drug sodium cromoglycate (Intal), in contrast, interacts with the mast cell surface and apparently prevents the in-rush of calcium ions, even if an allergen–antibody interaction occurs. Like most of the other compounds discussed in this chapter, it had its origins in folk medicine, and like penicillin was the product of a chance discovery.

The toothpick plant, *Ammi visnaga*, is indigenous to the Middle East, and has since biblical times been used in the treatment of respiratory problems. In 1879 one of its major constituents was isolated in crystalline form and given the name khellin. Its chemical structure was not elucidated until 1938, and in the meantime it had been shown to have a relaxant effect on various types of smooth muscle, like that in the gut.

In the mid-1950s, a small British pharmaceutical company called Bengers initiated a search for novel bronchodilators. They took khellin as their starting point and prepared a large number of structural derivatives. One of the major problems with any programme of this kind is the pharmacological evaluation of the compounds. This problem is especially acute for potential anti-asthma drugs, since there is no good animal model of asthma. A very neat solution was provided by Bengers' medical liaison officer, Roger Altounyan: he became the human guinea-pig for Bengers' new compounds.

Altounyan was a severe asthmatic and guinea-pig fur was an allergen for him, so he used to prepare a broth of the fur and then inhale the vapours. This caused bronchoconstriction in a reproducible fashion, and he could then take Bengers' putative bronchhodilators in order to test their efficacy. Many of the early compounds were water-insoluble or caused nausea, and to circumvent this problem the chemists prepared a range of analogues that could be inhaled as aerosol sprays. Eventually, in 1963, Altounyan made the chance discovery that, if he used an aerosol preparation of certain of these compounds ten minutes before inhaling his guinea-pig broth, they had a protective effect rather than a bronchodilator effect.

By now the management of Bengers had tired of this fruitless search for new bronchodilators and the programme was officially terminated. However, Altounyan and the main chemist on the project, Colin Fitzmaurice, continued to work in secret, and, when Bengers was taken over by Fisons in 1964, their project was reinstated. Finally, in 1964 they produced an analogue that appeared to have a long duration of action as a protective agent, but when they prepared a second batch of this new compound for further evaluation they could not reproduce its effects. This mystery was solved when it was discovered that an impurity in the original batch had the protective activity, and not the compound they were preparing. The impurity was subsequently shown to be a bis-chromone, sodium cromoglycate (Intal), and this had a protective effect even if administered four to six hours before allergen exposure.

One final problem had to be solved, and this was the means of delivery of the drug. It was poorly absorbed via the gastrointestinal tract, so it was necessary to inhale several milligrams in order to achieve a reasonable duration of protection. The solution came with the invention of the

Spinhaler, said to have been inspired by Altounyan's memories of his war years behind a Spitfire propeller. Intal powder is placed in the central compartment of the Spinhaler, and, as the patient breathes in, a tiny turbine at the mouth of the apparatus is caused to rotate and blows the drug deep into the lungs.

Although Intal is only effective as a protective agent for those suffering from allergic asthma, this does represent a major proportion of sufferers. Numerous other drugs have been evaluated since 1965, but none has been superior to sodium cromoglycate. One problem all other companies face is that they do not have Roger Altounyan as a human guinea-pig!

Drugs affecting the gastrointestinal tract

Plant extracts have been in use for thousands of years as purgatives, emetics, anti-emetics, and appetite enhancers, and as treatments for indigestion, diarrhoea, and gastric ulcers. Many of these extracts are still in use and are freely available in pharmacies and health food stores.

Purgatives and antidiarrhoeals

The ancient Egyptians used castor oil and beer according to the advice given in the Ebers papyrus: 'Berries of the castor oil tree, chew and swallow down with beer in order to clear out all that is in the body.' The Pharaohs preferred to use senna, which is in reality a collective name for extracts from various *Cassia* species, notably *C. senna*, *C. acutifolia*, and *C. angustifolia*. These contain an intestinal irritant called emodin, and this acts by stimulating the rhythmic, wave-like muscular contractions (peristalsis) that facilitate the passage of food through the gastrointestinal tract. The Greeks and Romans used the plant *Aloe barbadensis*. Juice from the leaves of this plant also contains emodin, as does Chinese rhubarb, *Rheum palmatum*. This last plant was once the main treatment for acute bacillary dysentery, especially by the British colonizers of Africa. They dosed themselves with powdered rhubarb until the diarrhoea and other symptoms subsided. As Dr R. W. Burkitt stated in the *Lancet* of September 1921, 'I know of no remedy in medicine which has such a magical effect. No one who has ever used rhubarb would dream of using anything else. I hope others will try it in this dreadful tropical scourge.'

The modes of action of the two main classes of purgative are thus lubrication (castor oil, olive oil, and liquid paraffin) or irritation (senna and aloes). These plants and the habit of purging were introduced into Europe by the Arabs during the ninth and tenth centuries, and by the seventeenth century twice-monthly purging was common in Britain. In the Americas cascara buckthorn (*Rhamnus purshiana*) was the plant of choice. The *conquistadores* were so impressed by the mildness and efficacy of its extracts that they christened it 'holy bark' (cascara), and the European settlers learnt of it from the Indians. It is still widely available and much used in the USA, though the bitter taste of its constituents (emodin and other similar compounds) necessitates the use of sugar-coated or chocolate-coated pills.

Another plant that contains emodin, *Aloe vera*, also has a long history of use, especially as a treatment for constipation. An old Chinese remedy known as *geng yi wan* (bathroom pills), is still in use today and comprises *Aloe vera*, mercury salts, and starch, in the ratio 4:3:3.

Once purging had started, it was often necessary to bring it to a halt, and in addition the poor sanitation of earlier epochs ensured that anti-diarrhoeal agents were in constant demand. The Ebers papyrus recommended a concoction made from figs, grapes, bread-dough, pit-corn, fresh lead-earth, onions, and elderberry, which seems more likely to cause diarrhoea than suppress it. But, as we saw in the section on opiates, the Egyptians were also aware of the gastrointestinal calmative properties of opium, and we use essentially the same treatment today in the form of kaolin and morphine. The morphine binds to opioid receptors in the gut and depresses peristalsis, and the slower movement of the intestinal contents allows an increased absorption of water to occur.

A whole host of other plants have been used over the centuries, including the fruit of the red cedar (*Juniperus virginiana*), the gum exuded by various *Pterocarpus* species, nutmeg, and various tannins. All of these extracts, including opium, treat the symptoms rather than the underlying causes. These are many and varied, and include bacterial or viral infections, food or chemical poisoning, and other conditions like ulcerative colitis, where there is probably an autoimmune component and malabsorption syndrome. Most of these conditions are now treated with wholly synthetic drugs, and their therapy owes nothing to folk medicine.

Emetics and anti-emetics

In the area of the brain known as the medulla oblongata there is a vomiting centre, which appears to receive electrical inputs from various other parts of the brain, from the gastrointestinal tract, and from pain receptors. A complex interplay of several neurotransmitters is probably involved, but acetylcholine, dopamine, and serotonin are major participants. The best natural emetic is without doubt ipecacuanha or ipecac from the South American plant *Cephaelis acuminata*. This has been in use for centuries and is still widely used in hospital casualty departments for the treatment of cases of poisoning in children and sometimes adults. The active constituents are emetine and cephaeline, which exert their effects through activation of the vomiting centre, but also through local irritation in the stomach. Squill, which was mentioned in the section on cardioactive drugs, has similar properties to ipecac.

There are many causes of emesis, including motion sickness, the so-called 'morning sickness' of the early weeks of pregnancy, and that due to gastrointestinal irritation. Historically, sickness was treated with various extracts of mint species, e.g. of *Mentha piperita* (peppermint), and with ginger root (*Zingiber officinale*). The effectiveness of the last extract for the treatment of motion sickness has been confirmed recently by experiment.

The most widely prescribed anti-emetic drugs are the wholly synthetic phenothiazines, but hyoscine, discussed in earlier chapters, is also effective for some conditions, as is metoclopramide, a dopamine antagonist. The involvement of histamine-responsive neurons in the causation of emesis is likely given the efficacy of antihistamines at least for travel sickness, although their tendency to induce drowsiness is a marked disadvantage for the driver. Finally, a new drug from Glaxo called ondansetron (Zofran) has potent anti-emetic activity and appears to act as an inhibitor of certain neurons in the gastrointestinal tract and the brain that are sensitive to 5-hydroxytryptamine (serotonin). It is likely to be particularly useful in the treatment of sickness induced by anticancer agents. Many of these appear to trigger release of serotonin in the gut, and this activates the vagal axons that terminate in the area postrema, a part of the oblongata medullary region in the brain particularly associated with control of emesis. Ondansetron is a potent inhibitor of a particular class of 5-hydroxytryptamine receptors (5-HT_3) on vagal nerve-endings and in the brain.

Flatulence, indigestion, and anti-ulcer drugs

Flatulence is caused by excessive gas in the stomach and intestine. The gas is mainly air, but may also comprise products of food decomposition, like hydrogen sulphide and methane. Many of the aromatic shrubs like tansy, fennel, dill, rosemary, anise, and the mints, as well as spices like cardamom, nutmeg, cloves, ginger, and cinnamon, have a long association with the treatment of flatulence. Culpeper said of the tansy (*Tanacetum vulgare*): 'It is also very profitable to dissolve and expel wind in the stomach, belly, or bowels, to procure women's courses, and expel windiness in the matrix.' And both he and Gerard were particularly enthusiastic about fennel (*Foeniculum vulgare*). Culpeper claimed that 'fennel is good to break wind ... [it] stays the hiccup, and takes away the loathings which oftentimes happen to the stomachs of sick and feverish persons'. Gerard, in his own inimitable style, stated that 'Fennel seede drunke, assuageth the paine of the stomache, and the wambling of the same, or desire to vomite, and breaketh winde'. The various constituents of the so-called carminatives probably act through a mild irritation of the gastrointestinal tract, and by stimulating minor movements that generate a belch.

Indigestion is most often caused by excess gastric acid, and remedies like sodium bicarbonate, calcium carbonate, aluminium hydroxide, and magnesium hydroxide (Milk of Magnesia) act by neutralizing this acid. The herbals recommended a variety of other preparations, but many of these were both exotic and ineffective. For example, the Ebers papyrus mentioned the use of onions cooked in sweet beer, and crushed hog's tooth taken in conjunction with a sugar cake. Dioscorides extolled the virtues of iron rust: 'Iron made burning hot, quenched in water, or wine, and drank, is good for ye coeliacall, dysenterical, splenicall, cholericall and for a dissolved stomach.'

The secretion of gastric acid is under the control of the autonomic nervous system, and many kinds of stimuli can initiate its release. These include the sight, smell, taste, and even the thought of food. The vagus nerve innervates much of the stomach and small intestine and controls the release of acetylcholine. Stimulation of certain cells at the lower end of the stomach initiate the release of a peptide hormone called gastrin, and once food is actually present in the stomach this too leads to the release of gastrin. In addition, histamine is also involved, and all three substances act upon the so-called parietal cells and stimulate the release of hydrochloric acid.

Hyperacidity can be caused by changes in the delicate balance of the two neurotransmitters, and an acute attack may be simply due to an emotional disturbance before a meal. Chronic hyperacidity is more often due to localized damage caused by drugs like aspirin or alcohol. These damage the mucous membranes that line the gut wall and protect it against the damaging effects of gastric acid and the digestive juices. The gut wall thus becomes susceptible to damage and the consequent formation of a gastric or duodenal ulcer. Something like 10–20 per cent of people in the West suffer from a peptic ulcer at some stage of their lives, and the treatment of this condition has long been of interest to the medical fraternity.

The most popular and successful folk medicine was liquorice root from the plant *Glycyrrhiza glabra*. Its active ingredient is glycyrrhizin, a derivative of glycyrrhetinic acid. This has a structure that partially resembles the mineralocorticoids, and as well as possessing healing potential it may cause sodium retention and potassium deficiency. Liquorice is probably the most often prescribed plant in Chinese herbal medicine, and a modern remedy for peptic ulcer involves administration of daily doses of up to 15 g of powdered liquorice root. Another remedy involves chewing tobacco soaked in a liquorice extract. In hospitals a semi-synthetic derivative of glycyrrhetinic acid, carbenoxolone sodium, was formerly used because this lacks the mineralocorticoid activity of glycyrrhizin while retaining the healing properties. It is believed to act by enhancing secretion of gastric mucus, thus protecting the ulcer from the damaging effects of the digestive enzymes.

The involvement of histamine prompted research in the 1960s directed towards the rational design of histamine antagonists. The known antihistamines, which were effective in allergic states, were totally ineffective for the treatment of peptic ulcers, and this led to the identification of two main classes of histamine receptors. These are the H_1 receptors in the lungs and upper respiratory tract, and H_2 receptors in the gut. Research initiated by Sir James Black and Robin Ganellin at Smith, Kline & French in 1965 led ultimately to the discovery of the potent H_2 antagonist cimetidine (Tagamet). Their strategy was to prepare compounds which resembled histamine but which possessed other structural features that would allow them to bind more strongly to the receptor, thus denying access to histamine. It was also vital that they did not trigger release of acid. After ten years of painstaking work, they realized their goal, and cimetidine entered clinical use in the UK in 1976, and a year later in the USA. By 1983 total world sales had reached £1 billion.

The drug is orally active, and at a dose of around 1 g per day, it relieves the symptoms of peptic ulcer and promotes healing. Later Glaxo produced its own variant of cimetidine, the even more potent ranitidine (Zantac), and this soon became Glaxo's number one selling drug, worth £1.7 billion in 1989.

The development of cimetidine is notable, because it was one of the first examples of rational drug design. The research group at SKF tried to produce a structural analogue of histamine that would mimic its physical and chemical properties under the physiological conditions present in the stomach. More recently, with the advent of computer-assisted molecular modelling, and a greater knowledge of the actual three-dimensional structure of the H_2 receptor, it has become possible to verify how the drug fits into the actual receptor. Most present drug design uses this facility, rather than the inspired guesswork of Black, Ganellin, and their co-workers.

These major advances have led to healing rates with the two drugs of around 85–90 per cent after a month or so. However, liquorice root, the mainstay of Chinese folk medicine, is likely to provide a cheap and effective alternative to the relatively expensive synthetic drugs in those countries that cannot afford them.

Antiparasitic agents

Man has always coexisted with parasites, and has been particularly troubled by the various parasitic worms (e.g. tapeworms), the arthropods (e.g. lice), and protozoa (e.g. the *Plasmodia* which cause malaria). The folk remedies are certainly more numerous than the conditions they were meant to treat. In the Ebers papyrus castor oil is mentioned frequently, but 'flesh-of-a-live-cow combined with freshly-baked bread, incense, lettuce, and sweet beer' was also prescribed.

Both Gerard and Culpeper had their own herb gardens, and although many of the plant species were grown specifically for their medicinal properties others had culinary importance. It must be remembered that before the advent of modern farming methods, which provide livestock with winter feedstuffs (e.g. turnips and swedes), all cattle were slaughtered in November and the meat salted. Inevitably this meant that when the meat was eventually cooked it was either very salty or putrid. To disguise these tastes our medieval forebears used large amounts of herbs and spices, especially pepper and cloves. Other spices, like cinnamon, nutmeg, ginger, cardamom, and mace, were also much in demand. In addition, perfumery materials, including camphor, sandalwood, and incense, were very popular, not only to mask the malodorous environment in which people lived, but also because it was believed that the vapours somehow afforded protection from malaria. The herbs and spices in the medieval diet certainly helped to keep parasitic infections under control. Their constituent terpenes, like menthol, carvone, and thujone, or phenols, like eugenol and myristicin, either caused paralysis of the worms or disrupted their life cycles.

The great majority of these spices and perfumes had to be imported from the Far East, and for many centuries the ports of Genoa and Venice had a monopoly of this trade. The commodities were carried by Chinese junk to Malaya, thence by Arab dhow to India, East Africa, Persia, and Arabia, and finally via the Red Sea or Persian Gulf into the Mediterranean area. The price differential between the Far Eastern traders and the merchants of Venice and Genoa was typically fiftyfold.

The Portuguese were the first to break the stranglehold of the great Italian ports, and their new empire in the Far East supplied Europe with spices and perfumes via the port of Lisbon. It was with the intention of breaking this new monopoly that Christopher Columbus embarked upon his voyages of discovery. He failed to find a new route to the East, but discovered the Americas instead. These new lands supplied exotic plants like tobacco, coffee, cocoa, coca, the potato, and cinchona; this last plant was to have the most profound effect upon the health of the peoples of the world.

At the time of these discoveries malaria was endemic in just about the whole of the known world. It has probably always been endemic in the Far East and Africa, but in the cooler, temperate regions it may have been relatively unknown in its most serious forms until around 500 BC. In order to understand this somewhat surprising suggestion, it is necessary to understand something of the life cycle of the malaria parasite and its insect host, the *Anopheles* mosquito (Fig. 4.13).

When an infected mosquito bites a human, it injects a small amount of saliva which contains an anticoagulant and the *Plasmodium* parasites. These are in the form of small, spindle-shaped cells, known as sporozoites, which migrate to the liver, colonize liver cells, and gradually coalesce. After five to fifteen days, the liver cells burst and release thousands of small cells known as merozoites, and these infect red blood cells (erythrocytes) or recolonize the liver. The merozoites grow in the erythrocytes until these have been completely overwhelmed. They then burst and release merozoites, which invade other erythrocytes, and pyrogens (chemical mediators of fever). The resultant bouts of fever occur every forty-eight hours in tertian malaria, every thirty-six hours in subtertian malaria, and every seventy-two hours in quartan malaria. These periods represent the times between infection and breakdown of the red blood cells, and are dependent upon the strains of parasites involved. The milder forms of malaria are due to *Plasmodium vivax* (tertian) and *P. malariae* (quartan), and the most serious form is due to *P. falciparum* (subtertian). The severity of the disease caused by this last organism is due to the fact that it can invade all types of red blood cells, both developing cells (reticulocytes) and mature erythrocytes. The other strains of parasites invade primarily one form or the other. The level of parasitism is thus much higher with *P. falciparum*, and it is common for the febrile condition to be essentially continuous rather than truly subtertian.

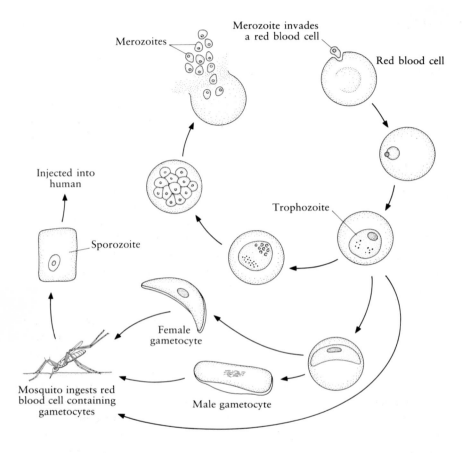

Fig. 4.13 The life cycle of the malaria parasite.

Some of the merozoites which enter the blood cells do not grow but undergo sexual differentiation into male and female gametocytes. When the human host is bitten by another mosquito, it is these gametocytes that fuse in the gut wall of the mosquito to produce new sporozoites.

The characteristic symptoms of malaria involve initial chills followed by high fever and ultimately a sweating stage. The disease is often highly debilitating, not only because of the recurrent bouts of fever, but also because of the anaemia caused by destruction of the red blood cells. In addition, the erythrocyte debris produced by infection with *P. falciparum* may block blood capillaries in the brain, with resultant convulsions and death. This malignant form of malaria has only been a problem in Europe in comparatively recent times.

Malaria probably reached southern Europe via the Nile valley, but fortunately the major strains of European mosquitoes, especially *Anopheles atroparvus*, were (and are) relatively refractory with regard to infection with *Plasmodium* parasites. The most susceptible strains of mosquito are *A. labranchiae* and *A. sacharevi*, and these were initially confined to the southern margins of Europe and to North Africa. Certainly there is no evidence that epidemics of malaria were a major cause of death in ancient times.

Hippocrates, who wrote on medicine in the fifth century BC, described forty-two case histories of persons suffering from fevers, but none of them appears to have suffered from malignant malaria. In contrast, Celsus in his *De Medicina*, written five centuries later, clearly describes the more fulminant form of malaria ('alterum longe perniciosius'), with bouts of fever lasting as long as thirty-six hours ('sex et triginta per accessionem occupat'). The paroxysms are also eloquently described: 'horrorem, ubi corpus totum intremit'.

Thus, it appears that infections with *P. falciparum* occurred in the time of Christ, but less frequently, if at all, in earlier times. This would explain how the vast armies of that period were able to travel large distances and wage war relatively efficiently without incurring huge losses from malaria. A good example of this is provided by the campaigns of Augustus in 31 BC, leading to the defeat of the combined armies and navies of Antony and Cleopatra. Over 90 000 soldiers and 150 000 naval personnel were employed by Augustus during the summer and autumn of that year, with much of the campaigning in North Africa; yet no significant losses from the disease were recorded. This can be compared with the 500 000 cases of malaria suffered by the British and Commonwealth forces during World War I, many cases of the disease being contracted in Greece and the Middle East.

The spread of malaria from North Africa through Europe can be traced to the large increases in population that occurred in Roman times. The resultant deforestation provided breeding grounds for the more susceptible strains of mosquitoes. Voluntary and enforced movements of populations encouraged the spread of the disease, as did the frequent upheavals caused by barbarian invasions. There were epidemics of malaria in the fifth century AD, as the Roman Empire crumbled, with subsequent neglect of good farming and irrigation practices, and more recently during the Industrial Revolution, when there was a mass exodus from the relatively healthy countryside to the squalid towns and cities.

All of the famous herbalists had their cures for the 'ague', and both Culpeper and Gerard strongly recommended St John's Wort, *Hypericum tomentosum*. Gerard merely repeated Disocorides' advice: '[Dioscorides] saith, that being drunk with wine, [St John's Wort] taketh away tertian and quartan agues.' Culpeper was a little more explicit: 'It is under the celestial sign of Leo ... The decoction of the leaves and seeds drank somewhat warm before the fits of ague, whether they be tertians or quartans, alters the fits, and ... doth take them quite away.'

There was, however, no effective treatment for malaria until the seventeenth century, when powdered bark from the South American cinchona tree was first introduced. The treatment was first mentioned by the monk Father Antonio de la Calaucha in the *Chronicle of St Augustine*, published in about 1633. He claimed that the bark of a tree growing in the part of the Inca Empire known as Quito (now Ecuador) would cure malaria. He wrote: 'A tree grows which they call the fever tree in the country of Loxa ... When made into a powder amounting to the size of two small silver coins and given as a beverage, it cures the fevers and tertians.' The Incas called the tree *quina*, and although there is no evidence that they knew of its medicinal value, they may have been keeping it a secret from the *conquistadores*. It was left to the Jesuit missionaries to organize the collection of the bark and its shipment to Europe. Not surprisingly it became known as 'Jesuit's powder'.

The Jesuit Cardinal Johannes de Lugo did much to popularize its use, especially in Rome, where malaria was rampant. The name, in fact, derives from the Italian *mal'aria* (bad air), which also reflects the supposed origin of the ague. It was not at all uncommon for cardinals and their attendants to contract malaria en route to papal gatherings at the Vatican. For example, the first Archbishop of Canterbury, St Augustine, died of marsh fever (probably malaria) in 587 while *en route* from Ostia to Rome. So Cardinal de Lugo had little trouble persuading the clerics and the citizens of Rome to take the exceptionally bitter powder.

However, like all new remedies, many physicians were sceptical, especially since it had been introduced by a religious order which was generally detested. Its eventual success was ensured by an Englishman, Robert Talbor. He had studied as an apprentice apothecary in Cambridge, and would certainly have learnt of the use of Jesuit's powder during his time in that city. A local physician, Robert Brady, was definitely prescribing the bark as early as 1660. Talbor moved to Essex in 1661 and began practising as a quack physician. Much of the county was at that time marshy and malaria was both endemic and prevalent. He quickly made a name for

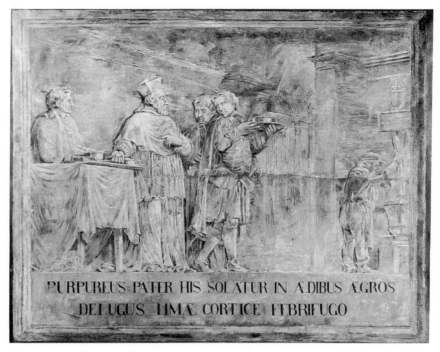

PURPUREUS PATER HIS SOLATUR IN ÆDIBUS ÆGROS
DELUGUS LIMÆ CORTICE FEBRIFUGO

Cardinal Johannes de Lugo did much to popularize the use of the powdered bark of the cinchona tree as a treatment for malaria. A seventeenth century engraving in the Ospele di Santo Spirito in Rome, reproduced in this anonymous twentieth century oil painting, illustrates the discovery and dissemination of the medicinal use of cinchona extracts. (Wellcome Institute Library, London.)

himself with a speciality drug for the treatment of the ague, though he never revealed what he was prescribing. To ensure success he wrote a book in 1672 entitled *Pyretologia: a Rational Account of the Cause and Cure of Agues*, and in this he warned of the dangers of other preparations: 'all palliative cures . . . especially Jesuit's powder, for I have seen most dangerous effects follow the taking of that medicine'.

Much to the annoyance of the Royal College of Physicians, Charles II appointed him court physician in 1678, and had cause to be grateful when Talbor cured him of a bout of tertian fever one year later. But Talbor's career reached its pinnacle in France, where he cured Louis XIV's son, the Dauphin, not to mention other European aristocrats. He still refused to reveal the secret of his remedy, but agreed in 1681 to a lucrative arrangement with Louis that assured him a pension for life, and a revelation of the recipe following his death. He died the next year and his secret was revealed as nothing other than a mixture of Jesuit's powder and wine. This was precisely the brew that was already prescribed by Thomas Sydenham, who also wrote extensively and perceptively about the ague and its cure. Of the cause he wrote: 'When insects do swarm extraordinarily and when fevers and agues (especially quartans) appears early as about midsummer, then autumn proves very sickly.' His description of the symptoms was very precise: 'All agues begin with shiverings and rigours, succeeded by heat and terminated by sweats ... Soon or late ... the paroxysm repeats its attack, the intervals being ... for the quotidian twenty-four hours, for the tertian eight and forty ... etc.' And his remedies would have ensured an alcoholic haze at the very least: 'You may mix an ounce of bark with two pints of claret and give it ... in doses of eight or nine spoonsful.'

By now the religious bigotries of earlier years had receded, and cinchona bark became accepted world-wide. A new controversy now arose over the mode of administration of the drug. It was widely believed that the mode of action of the drug was as a nerve tonic, and during the eighteenth century cinchona preparations were used for a whole range of conditions. This led not only to inappropriate prescribing but also to gross over-prescribing when the initial doses failed to achieve the desired remissions. Interestingly, this drug abuse provided the inspiration for the German physician, Samuel Hahnemann's regimen of drug therapy that ultimately became homoeopathic medicine. Hahnemann apparently took a large dose of cinchona bark in 1796, and perhaps not surprisingly he suffered paroxysms similar to those experienced with malaria. He reasoned that minute doses of a drug that caused a condition should be used to effect a cure, and proceeded to test his theory using human volunteers and around ninety preparations. The modern practice of homoeopathic medicine embraces most of his findings and uses, for example, minute doses of arsenic for the treatment of gastroenteritis and food poisoning, or can-tharidin (Spanish fly) for urinary tract conditions. These are precisely the symptoms that would be caused by a larger dose of the 'drugs'. Whatever the value of Hahnemann's new methods, they at least spared his patients from the overdoses prescribed by other physicians.

Despite the growing popularity of cinchona in the eighteenth century, its origins were obscure until specimens were obtained and classified by the Swedish botanist Carl Linné (Linnaeus). He assigned the tree to a new family, which he christened *Cinchona*. The derivation of the name has been often ascribed to the Count of Chinchón, then Spanish viceroy in Peru, but more probably to the Indian name for the tree.

The active principle, quinine, was not isolated in pure form until 1820, and the two French chemists involved in this isolation, Pelletier and Caventou, went on to produce vast quantities of quinine in their Paris factories. The clinical efficacy of the pure drug was quickly demonstrated, and the demand for cinchona bark soon outstripped the supply. In an early example of what would now be described as 'rape of the rain forest', collectors carried out wholesale stripping of cinchona trees, which were then left to die.

The Dutch botanist J. C. Hasskarl mounted an expedition in 1852 to gather seeds for a planting in the Dutch colonies on Java. In 1852 he dispatched 500 plants by fast warship, but only seventy-five survived the journey, and these failed to thrive on the volcanic slopes in Java. Further efforts over the years to 1863 resulted in a total stock of 208 322 seeds, 612 770 plants in nurseries, and 539 040 in permanent sites, but most of the trees yielded a very low percentage of quinine. The famous British explorer Richard Spruce and his companion Charles Markham managed to procure 100 000 seeds, but despite repeated efforts in British India and Ceylon, the resultant trees also gave a low yield. The whole venture was so unprofitable that a million cinchona trees had to be destroyed in 1900. Ultimately the Dutch did succeed in producing a high-yielding strain, but this was more by luck than through a careful breeding programme. A British settler in Peru, Charles Ledger, obtained the seeds of a particularly good strain via his Indian servant, and some of these seeds eventually turned up in Java. The resultant trees, subsequently christened *Cinchona ledgeriana*, were able to yield bark with as much as 10 per cent quinine, and this led to the Dutch capturing a world-wide monopoly of quinine supply.

In the meantime a hesitant start was made in the determination of the mode of transmission of malaria. In 1880 the Frenchman Alphonse Laveran identified the presence of parasites in infected erythrocytes, and the Englishman Ronald Ross established the mosquito as the carrier in 1897. Other experiments were carried out by Patrick Manson and his collaborators in the marshy areas of the Roman Campagna. These studies were both brave and conclusive. In one, Manson obtained mosquitoes from Rome, infected them with a relatively benign form of tertian malaria, and then had them shipped to London. Once there, they were allowed to bite Manson's son and a laboratory assistant named George Warren, both of whom subsequently developed malaria.

The Dutch monopoly of quinine was finally broken by three events: the Japanese invasion of Java in 1942, the widespread use of DDT after the war to destroy mosquitoes in their breeding areas, and the introduction of wholly synthetic drugs like Paludrine. The sudden cessation of supplies in 1942 led to a large-scale effort in the USA and Britain to produce synthetic anti-malarials. The German company I. G. Farben had introduced mepacrine (Atebrin) in the 1930s, and this was the main drug produced and used by the allies. R. B. Woodward and W. E. Doering of Harvard reported a synthesis of quinine in 1944, but the route was too complex for industrial production. After the war, numerous analogues were made and tested, and proguanil (Paludrine) and pyrimethamine (Daraprim) have been highly effective.

As to the mode of action of quinine, it appears to have little effect on the sporozoites or on any stage before infection of the erythrocytes. In these it binds to the parasite's DNA, ultimately preventing the protein biosynthesis required for its growth. Just as with the bacteria, the various *Plasmodium* species have over the years developed resistance to quinine and to most of the synthetic drugs, and there is little chance of a vaccine in the foreseeable future. *Plasmodium falciparum* and its relatives are thus likely to remain formidable foes for many years to come. As for quinine, it is still produced in large quantities in Indonesia, and satisfies a tradition first instituted by the British Raj. As the sun went down, the colonizers of the Far East put gin into their Indian tonic water to disguise the bitter taste of the quinine. In today's gin and tonic, the quinine enhances the flavour of the gin!

This section has been primarily concerned with malaria and its treatment, and this reflects the importance of the disease and the historical pre-eminence of quinine as a naturally occurring antimalarial drug. Other parasitic infections are also of wide occurrence, and trypanosomiasis and amoebiasis merit some discussion.

Several species of trypanosomes occur in Africa and South America and, of these, three are pathogenic to man. In Africa *Trypanosoma gambiense* and *T. rhodesiense* are the causative pathogens of African sleeping sickness; and in South America *T. cruzi* causes South American trypanosomiasis, often known as Chagas' disease. The African form of sleeping sickness is more severe and results from the bite of an infected tsetse fly. When the parasites enter the brain they cause meningoencephalitis, leading to lethargy, coma, and death. The South American form produces chronic debilitation rather than a rapid death. The trypanosomes infect most tissues, thus producing intermittent fever, enlargement of the liver and spleen, and sometimes encephalitis. A small green beetle, *Triatoma megista*, which lives in the mud walls of houses, is the vector of this form of trypanosomiasis, and in parts of Brazil the incidence of the disease is as high as 20 per cent of the population. It has been suggested that Charles Darwin was infected during his South American sojourn, and certainly his frequent bouts of lethargy in later life would be consistent with this theory.

Amoebic dysentery is common almost world-wide, and is caused by infection with the parasite *Entamoeba histolytica*. Poor sanitation and inadequate food hygiene are usually blamed for the spread of the disease, and something approaching 10 per cent of the world's population are probably affected. The main symptom is acute or chronic diarrhoea, and for centuries in Brazil this has been treated by the administration of ipecacuanha. The efficacy of the major constituent, emetine, was first established in 1912 and provides a further example of a folk remedy with useful clinical utility.

Much effort continues to identify plant extracts that have amoebicidal, trypanosomal, or anti-malarial activity, and one plant is of particular contemporary interest. Extracts of the plant *Artemesia annua* have been valued for centuries in China for their antimalarial activity. As early as AD 340 the Chinese herbalist Ge Hong claimed that fevers could be treated by drinking a concoction of one handful of *qing hao* in a litre of water. Initial attempts in the 1970s to establish the biological efficacy of the plant extracts were disappointing, but in 1972 Chinese workers managed to isolate the major active ingredient which they named *qinghaosu*, or artemisinin. Its structure was finally elucidated in 1980, and it has considerable potency in inhibiting the growth of primaquine-resistant *Plasmodium falciparum*. It is also surprisingly non-toxic, with median lethal doses for mice and rats of around 4 and 5 g per kilogram respectively. This encouraged the Chinese to begin a clinical trial, and by 1979 they had treated 2099 cases of malaria with clinical cures in every case. Although the mode of action is presently unknown, several studies are underway to try to optimize the antimalarial activity of *qinghaosu* through the synthesis of more potent analogues. This work is particularly exciting, because it offers the promise of a rationally designed antiparasitic drug based upon a natural model. This was never achieved with quinine.

Anticancer agents

Parasitic diseases are the scourge of the Third World, but cancer is the most feared disease in the developed countries. Almost three million new cases are diagnosed each year in the West. Current statistics for the UK suggest that one in three people are affected by cancer at some stage in their lives, and 20–25 per cent of deaths are due to the condition.

The actual cause of a particular cancer is usually unknown, but invariably involves one or more factors. These include exposure to a carcinogen, an oncogenic virus, a parasite, radiation, or physical trauma, in conjunction with an inherited genetic disposition towards the disease or an age-related breakdown of the immune surveillance mechanisms. The carcinogenicity of certain chemicals is well established, such as the benzpyrenes in cigarette smoke or chimney soot, chromium salts in industrial waste, and nitrosamines or mycotoxins in the diet. Such environmental factors are probably responsible for the majority of cancers, and certainly explain the vast differences in incidence rates between localities or peoples. In the nineteenth century chimney sweeps contracted scrotal cancer because of exposure to chimney soot. People in the Honan province of China have a high incidence of oesophageal cancer, while in parts of Mozambique there is a high incidence of liver cancer: both of these trends can be ascribed in part to mycotoxins in the diet. The 200-fold difference between the incidences of skin cancer in Queensland, Australia, and in India is presumably due to the high levels of ultraviolet radiation falling upon the fair skins of European immigrants. In addition, the higher incidences of colon and breast cancers in the West compared with those in Japan are probably attributable to differences in the intake of dietary fats. In contrast, Japan has the highest incidence of stomach cancer in the world, and this has been blamed on their high intake of salted fish and a lack of fresh fruit and vegetables. This latter deficiency is of particular interest, since an increasing body of evidence indicates a protective effect for the vitamins A, C, and E, and the trace element selenium, all common in fruit and vegetables.

The role of viruses is harder to determine, but it is estimated that viruses contribute to development of around 20 per cent of female tumours and 8 per cent of male tumours. Hepatitis B virus is certainly implicated in the cause of primary liver cancer, and in parts of Africa the Epstein–Barr virus is associated with the prevalence of Burkitt's lymphoma. This virus is also responsible for glandular fever (infectious mononucleosis) and plays a part in the cause of oesophageal cancer in China. Their mode of action is now partially understood and involves an initial infection, often early in life, with subsequent incorporation of the viral DNA into the host cell DNA, where it lies dormant (repressed) for many years. Later in life, usually at a time when the person's resistance has been lowered due to illness or the ravages of time, the viral DNA is derepressed and produces multiple copies of enzymes that disrupt the cellular control mechanisms.

A more insidious sequence of events was first demonstrated in 1980, when it was established that certain constituent genes of normal cells, so-called oncogenes, have a propensity to become activated following mutation or some other event. It is probable that these genes have an essential role during fetal development or other stages of early life, when rapid growth and differentiation is required, but are then repressed. Once de-repressed, these oncogenes code for the production of proteins that overcome the usual cellular control mechanisms. The rogue cells then reproduce themselves without constraint.

Possible mechanisms for this escape from regulation have been proposed. It appears that most cells produce factors that control the growth of other cells, but do not manufacture self-regulatory products. The oncogene and viral products include growth factors for the parent cell or deviant growth factor receptors that are in a permanent state of activation.

Unregulated growth is thus one of the main characteristics of a cancer cell, together with its ability to avoid recognition as a foreign cell by the body's immune surveillance mechanisms. Contrary to popular belief cancer cells do not necessarily reproduce any more rapidly than normal cells: they merely grow without constraint. More insidiously they also have the propensity to break away from their primary growth site (primary tumour) and metastasize to other sites, where they produce secondary tumours. It is these metastases in the lungs, brain, liver, or bones that are the prime cause of pain, debility, and ultimately death.

In the past the initial treatment for cancer was usually surgery, and this still remains a major option for many cancers. However, by the time a tumour is visible by X-ray investigation or by physical examination (palpable), it will usually have a diameter of 1 cm and constitute one billion cells. It may also have spread to other far-distant sites. Surgery and the more recently invented techniques of radiotherapy are thus of limited, local benefit, and until the advent of chemotherapy there was little that could be done to eliminate metastases.

The era of cancer chemotherapy could perhaps be dated from 1865, when Lissauer gave Fowler's solution (potassium arsenite) to a patient suffering from leukaemia, with positive results. More realistically the modern use of cancer chemotherapeutic agents began in 1942, when Dougherty, Gilman, Goodman, and Lindskog initiated a clinical trial with a nitrogen mustard. The nitrogen mustards were developed as successors to the sulphur mustards, like mustard gas, which were used as blistering agents during World War I. These second-generation agents of chemical warfare were originally destined for use in World War II, but neither the

Germans nor the Allies dared use them. A wartime embargo on scientific publications meant that the clinical work of Dougherty and co-workers was not published until 1946, but since then the nitrogen mustards have been widely used as effective, though highly toxic, antitumour agents. Of more direct relevance to this book are the natural plant products that have been used in cancer chemotherapy. Like the nitrogen mustards they exert their antitumour effects through inhibition of cell division.

It has been estimated that around 35 billion cells divide each day in a healthy adult, and any of these divisions could produce a rogue cell population that continues to grow without constraint. Not all tumours grow rapidly, and a typical lung carcinoma doubles in size every ninety days, while a colon carcinoma takes eighty days for the same increase in size. In contrast, a lymphoma may double in size every three to four days, and a testicular teratoma takes five to six days. These differences are reflected in the relative ease of controlling these tumours with drugs. The fast-growing tumours can usually be completely eradicated if treated early enough, while lung and colon carcinomas are usually refractory to chemotherapy.

The key to the successful use of anticancer drugs is a knowledge of their modes of inhibition of cell division. The cell cycle is divided into several phases: the S phase, during which DNA synthesis occurs; a resting phase, the so-called premitotic interval (G2); cell division or mitosis; and a post-mitotic resting phase (G1). The cell is most susceptible to damage during the phase of synthesis and during mitosis. Many anticancer drugs damage DNA or form chemical bonds with it, thus preventing the DNA double helix from unwinding and reproducing itself. Other drugs interfere with the synthesis or assembly of the protein tubulin. This is the major constituent of the numerous microtubules (fibres rather like the spokes of an umbrella: see Fig. 4.14) that provide the mitotic spindle during cell division. Many plant-derived anticancer agents act via this mechanism, and, of these, colchicine, podophyllotoxin, and the vinca alkaloids have the closest associations with folk medicine.

The autumn crocus, *Colchicum autumnale*, was much prized in Roman times as a treatment for gout. This is a condition in which uric acid, a product of the breakdown of nucleic acids (the chemical constituents of DNA and RNA) accumulate due to inefficient excretion. Deposition of crystals of uric acid in the joints leads to an inflammatory state not un-like rheumatism. Byzantine physicians, and later on Arab physicians, prescribed extracts of the plant for both of these conditions. It was again highly popular in the eighteenth century, but it was only in the

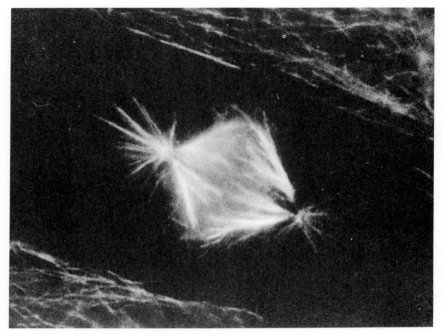

Fig. 4.14 Cell mitosis. The process has been visualized through the use of radioactive tracers and a photographic technique known as autoradiography.

twentieth century that the major constituent, colchicine, was shown to be cytotoxic.

Its mode of action in gout probably involves inhibition of migration of leukocytes which would normally mediate the inflammatory response to the crystals. The antitumour activity is a result of its ability to bind to tubulin and prevent polymerization of the protein to form new microtubules. Unfortunately, colchicine is too toxic for general clinical use, though it has been invaluable as an aid to understanding the mechanisms of inhibition of other cytotoxic drugs.

In the *Leech Book* of Bald (*c.* AD 950) an extract of the wild chervil, probably *Myrrhis odorata*, was mentioned as a salve for the treatment of tumours. The plant produces several lignans related in structure to the cytotoxic agent podophyllotoxin. Better sources of this type of compound include the Himalayan species *Podophyllum emodii* and the North American species *Podophyllum peltatum*, or American may-apple. Extracts of the roots of these plants contain podophyllotoxin and α-peltatin as major constituents. The American Indians used the root extract primarily as a purgative, emetic, and poison (for suicide), though the Penobscott Indians in Maine are said to have used the extracts for the treatment of venereal warts. Tincture of podophyllum is still available as a proprietary treatment for skin warts and verrucas.

In 1942 Kaplan reported that venereal warts could indeed be cured by topical applications of podophyllum resin, and this demonstration encouraged Hartwell and co-workers at the National Cancer Institute in Washington to test the extracts on experimental animal tumours. Although podophyllotoxin had been isolated in pure form by Podwyssotzki in 1880, its structure was not elucidated until 1958 by Hartwell and Schrecker. Subsequent investigation showed that it bound to a site on tubulin very close to that occupied by colchicine, and that like this compound it was a powerful spindle poison. A few cancer patients were treated with podophyllotoxin or α-peltatin, but the minor improvements observed were outweighed by the serious accompanying gastrointestinal toxicity.

In 1954 the Sandoz company of Switzerland began a programme of research aimed at the synthesis of structural analogues with a better therapeutic index, i.e. an improved cell-killing potential (cytotoxicity) relative to general toxicity. A number of naturally occurring carbohydrate derivatives of the lignans had been isolated, and the Sandoz chemists took these as a starting point for their synthetic efforts. Of the numerous analogues prepared using podophyllotoxin as the starting material, two were particularly potent, and these were christened etoposide and teniposide. Clinical trials began in the early 1970s, and both compounds proved to be highly effective for the treatment of a number of cancers. Teniposide is especially useful in the treatment of refractory childhood leukaemia, while etoposide is the drug of choice for patients with small-cell lung cancer, a particularly aggressive and relatively fast-growing lung cancer.

Interestingly, despite the close structural similarities between these semi-synthetic analogues and podophyllotoxin, neither of them binds to tubulin or acts as a spindle poison. Instead, they bind to an enzyme called topoisomerase II and prevent it from assisting in the duplication of DNA during the S phase of the cell cycle. The enzyme has a dual role, which involves producing nicks in DNA strands and then rejoining the strands once duplication of the fragments has been achieved. Whatever the actual mechanism by which etoposide and teniposide act, the ultimate result of their association with topoisomerase II is the production of nicked DNA strands that are not repaired.

In contrast to *Colchicum autumnale* and the *Podophyllum* species, there is no mention in the folk literature of a use for the rosy periwinkle (*Catharanthus roseus* formerly *Vinca rosea*) in cancer chemotherapy. It was, however, used in the form of a tea by diabetics in the Philippines, South Africa, India, and Australia, and this encouraged R. L. Noble and his Canadian co-workers to screen extracts of the plant for hypoglycaemic activity. The extracts proved to be totally ineffective when tested on rabbits with artificially increased concentrations of blood glucose, but several of the animals died shortly afterwards from severe bacterial infections. This was shown to be due to a gross depletion of their white blood cells, with a consequent decrease in their ability to mount an immune response to invading organisms. Toxicity of this kind is a common adverse effect of treatment with cytotoxic drugs, and Noble's group went on to test the extracts on a number of animal tumours, with excellent results. They reported their findings in 1955 and were immediately approached by scientists from Eli Lilly, who had also been working with *C. roseus*. Thereafter the two groups pooled their resources and information.

Between 1960 and 1962 they identified four active alkaloids from the plant: vinblastine, vincristine, leurosidine, and leurosine. The biological screening was enormously facilitated by the availability of a mouse leukaemia P-1534 which was exquisitely sensitive to the drugs. At doses of less than 0.3 mg per kilogram given over a ten-day period, there were many long-term survivors among the leukaemic mice. Other animal tumours were equally responsive, and clinical trials on humans were soon under way.

Thirty years on, one can say without fear of contradiction that thousands of lives have been saved through the use of vincristine and vinblastine. The five-year survival prospects for patients with Hodgkin's disease was a depressing 5 per cent in 1970, but has now risen to 98 per cent with a regimen that includes vincristine, the antimetabolites methotrexate and 5-mercaptopurine, and the anti-inflammatory drug prednisolone. The comparable figures for acute lymphoblastic leukaemia in children are 5 and 60 per cent when they receive initial treatment with vincristine and prednisolone, followed by various other anticancer drugs and bone-marrow replacement. Finally, for testicular teratoma there was a spectacular increase in the number of complete cures following the introduction in the mid-1970s of vinblastine and the mould product bleomycin alternating with courses of the inorganic drug cisplatin, a platinum derivative. Well over 90 per cent of all teratoma patients now survive. These are all triumphs of combination chemotherapy.

The mode of action of the vinca alkaloids is similar to that of podophyl-lotoxin and colchicine, though they have a discrete binding site on tubulin. A number of analogues have been prepared, but only vindesine has signi-ficant value. Although the compounds can be prepared synthetically, the routes are long and expensive. In consequence, Eli Lilly processes around 8000 kg of flowers from *C. roseus* each year in order to satisfy the demand for the drugs.

The successes with plant extracts encouraged the Cancer Chemotherapy National Service Centre (CCNSC) at Bethesda near Washington to embark upon a major screening programme in 1955. This was an exten-sion of programmes begun by the Sloan Kettering Institute in New York and the CSIRO in Australia, both of which screened over 2000 plant species between 1945 and 1955. During the period from 1955 to 1980, the CCNSC screened a further half a million plant extracts and synthetic compounds, and a majority of today's anticancer drugs had their origins in this programme.

The new drugs were obtained from three natural sources: moulds, terrestrial plants, and more recently from marine organisms. The moulds have been a particularly rich source of clinically useful agents, and these include the bleomycins from *Streptomyces verticillus*, doxorubicin, an anthracycline, from *Streptomyces peucetius*, and the mitomycins from *Streptomyces verticillatus*. In addition, the cyclosporins from *Trichoderma inflatum*, although devoid of anticancer activity, are potent immuno-suppressants and are used to treat patients who have received bone-marrow transplants (and organ transplants).

Terrestrial plants have yielded the clinically effective maytansinoids (from *Maytenus serrata*), ellipticine and related compounds (from *Ochrosia elliptica*), as well as experimental drugs like taxol from the yew (*Taxus baccata*), the quassinoids like bruceantin from the family Simaroubaceae, and camptothecin from *Camptotheca accuminata*.

Marine organisms represent a relatively untapped source of interesting natural products, and during the last fifteen years the National Cancer Institute has screened thousands of marine plants and animals for biologic-ally interesting molecules. Among the compounds that are presently under evaluation, the cephalostatins from the marine worm *Cephalodiscus gil-christi* and the dolastatins from the sea-hare *Dolabella auricularia* have particularly potent cytotoxic activity.

These and other naturally occurring anticancer agents may have a major impact on cancer chemotherapy over the next few years, but it would be misleading to leave the impression that natural products are the only effective anticancer drugs. Numerous totally synthetic drugs are currently in use for the treatment of a whole range of cancers. For example, the drugs aminoglutethimide and tamoxifen are the most widely prescribed agents for the treatment of hormone-dependent breast cancer. About one-third of mammary cancers require a supply of oestrogens, the female sex hormones, for their continued growth, and aminoglutethimide inhibits the enzyme aromatase that assists in the production of these hormones. In contrast, tamoxifen binds to oestrogen receptors in the cytoplasm of the cell and denies access to oestrogens. This prevents the translocation of receptor–hormone complexes into the cell nucleus, where they would normally interact with DNA and initiate a burst of new cell growth. Both drugs thus prevent the growth of breast cancer cells.

As more information becomes available about the development and growth of cancer cells, it will be possible to design drugs that will interfere with particular stages of their life cycle. In the meantime the various screening programmes will continue to provide novel natural products for the treatment of a disease that will become more prevalent as life expectancy and environmental pollution both increase.

The future

The major screening programmes that were mentioned in the last section have continued to yield novel, biologically active molecules. Most of these have come from plants or microorganisms, and three recent discoveries will serve to highlight the continuing importance of this work.

In 1976 the mould metabolite compactin was isolated from *Penicillium citrinum* and from *P. brevicompactum*. Four years later the structurally similar fungal metabolite mevinolin was isolated from *Aspergillus terreus*. It was quickly established that both compounds could inhibit the biosynthesis of cholesterol, and since hypercholesterolaemia is a major risk factor for those with coronary artery disease, the clinical potential of these compounds was considerable. In the event the Merck, Sharp, and Dohme Co. have recently been given approval by the Federal Drug Administration in the USA to market mevinolin (Mevacor) for use in hypercholesterolaemic patients. It is too early to assess the impact of this therapy on the long-term survival of these patients, but the short-term effects have been highly encouraging.

During the 1960s a screening programme at the Central Drug Research Institute in Lucknow, India, paid special attention to plants that were used in Indian folk medicine. Plants of the species *Coleus* have an especially long history of use, and various extracts formed the basis of many old Vedic remedies for asthma, epilepsy, fever, colic, indigestion, piles, heart disease, etc. In present day India, tubers from the plant *Coleus barbatus* (*C. forskohli*) are used as constituents of various condiments, but in 1977 pharmacological evaluation of plant extracts indicated that other activities could be of interest. The major constituent, forskolin, was isolated and shown to have both antihypertensive activity and positive inotropic activity (it increases cardiac output). It produces these effects through activation of the enzyme adenylate cyclase, with consequent production of the intra-cellular second messenger cyclic AMP. Forskolin thus promises to be of interest both as a potential drug and also as an experimental tool for the investigation of intracellular signalling.

Finally, several plant-derived compounds show promise as inhibitors of the virus that causes AIDS (acquired immune deficiency syndrome). At the present time around 1–1.5 million Americans are carriers of the human immunodeficiency virus (HIV), and many more persons have been infected world-wide. Much is now known about the virus, which is one of a small group known as the retroviruses. It is thus unusual in having its genetic information in the form of RNA instead of DNA, and it uses this as a blueprint for the production of viral DNA, which is then incorporated into the host cell DNA. After infection, the virus binds preferentially to T4 lymphocytes, which are essential regulatory cells of the immune system. A glycoprotein (i.e. a protein that has short carbohydrate sequences attached at various points) called gp120 on the virus surface attaches to a glyco-protein called CD4 on the T4 lymphocyte. Subsequent fusion allows the virus to enter the cell where it uses one of its key enzymes, reverse tran-scriptase, to produce viral DNA (see Fig. 4.15).

The viral DNA is then incorporated into the host cell's DNA. Here it may lie dormant for many years, just like an oncogene, before being derepressed and providing the blueprint for viral protein and RNA manu-facture. As an increasing number of new virus particles are assembled, the T4 cells are weakened and may subsequently die. Consequent upon this gradual destruction of the T4 cell population, a state of immune deficiency is established, and the patient develops the classic symptoms of AIDS. Death is ultimately due to the effects of opportunistic infections or the effects of rare tumours like Kaposi's sarcoma.

Many drugs have been screened for activity, and although some like zidovudine (azidothymidine, AZT) and dideoxyinosine have clinical value, they only slow the progressive destruction of T4 cells. The best kind of treatment would be one that prevented the association of the virus with the

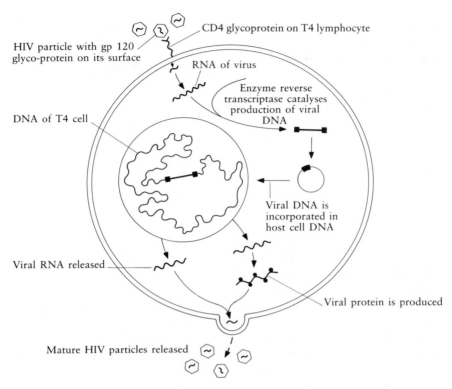

Fig. 4.15 Infection by the human immunodeficiency virus (HIV), and its replication within the cell.

CD4 receptors. There is now some hope that certain plant products may have this activity.

In the mid-1970s research groups in Belgium, Japan, Australia, and England reported, more or less simultaneously, the discovery of a number of novel natural products. All possessed structures that resembled the natural carbohydrates (e.g. glucose, mannose, fructose) but included in their rings a nitrogen atom in place of an oxygen atom (see Fig. 4.16). They were derived from such diverse species as the Japanese mulberry tree (*Morus* species), *Swainsona* species from Australia, and locoweeds (*Astragalus* species) from the western parts of the USA.

Of these compounds, deoxynojirimycin, swainsonine, and castanospermine (from *Castanospermum australe*) were the most intensely studied, and it was quickly established that they function as glycosidase inhibitors,

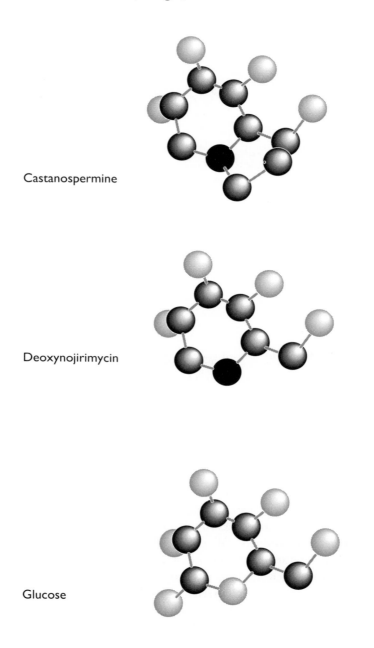

Castanospermine

Deoxynojirimycin

Glucose

Fig. 4.16 Comparison of the structures of castanospermine, deoxynojiro-mycin, and glucose.

that is, they interfere with the functions of various enzymes (glycosidases) that assist in the removal of carbohydrate residues from, for example, glycoproteins. This was of considerable interest, given the importance of glycoproteins as regulators of viral infectivity and the immune response and in the metastasis of cancer cells. Both castanospermine and swainsonine were subsequently shown to inhibit the growth of certain tumour cells, and the former compound also modifies the infectivity of HIV, probably by modifying the structure of its glycoprotein gp120. Not surprisingly, the synthesis and biological evaluation of analogues of these natural molecules is being pursued with great vigour.

These further examples of natural products as real or potential medicinal agents provide a salutary reminder of how much is still to be learnt about the existence and utility of naturally occurring substances. Our forebears experimented with plant extracts and discovered poisons, hallucinogens, and medicines. We can still do the same today—but for how much longer? It is likely that only a fraction of the plant species that exist in the rain forests have been investigated, yet these same forests are being destroyed at the rate of about 50 hectares every minute. There is no way of knowing how many potential drugs are being lost in this way, and of course our other environmental assaults on the planet transcend these serious losses. A character in the Gilbert and Sullivan opera *Ruddigore* claims that 'Man is Nature's sole mistake'; one might now add 'the destruction of Nature will be Man's last mistake'.

Bibliography

Introduction

Bowman, W. C. and Rand, M. J. (1980). *Textbook of Pharmacology* (2nd edn). Blackwell.

Rose, S. (1991). *The Chemistry of Life* (3rd edn). Penguin.

Murder

Akratanakul, P., Guillemin, J., Meselson, M., Nowicke, J. W., and Seeley, J. D. (1985). Yellow rain. *Sci. Am.* **253** (Sept.), 122.

Austwick, P. and Mattocks, R. (1979). Naturally occurring carcinogens in food. *Chem. Ind.* 76.

Bisset, N. G. (1989). Arrow and dart poisons. *J. Ethnopharmacol.* **25**, 1.

Blubaugh, L. V. and Linegar, C. R. (1948). Curare and modern medicine. *Econ. Bot.* **2**, 73.

Buchwald, H. D., Fischer, H. G., Fuhrman, F. A., and Mosher, H. S. (1984). Tarichatoxin-tetrodotoxin: A potent neurotoxin. *Science* **144**, 1100.

Campbell, W. A. (1990). Inorganic poisons: Vermilion and verdigris—not just pretty colours. *Chem. Brit.* **26**, 558.

Caporael, L. R. (1976). Ergotism: The Satan loosed in Salem. *Science* **192**, 21.

Catterall, W. A. (1980). Neurotoxins that act on voltage-sensitive sodium channels in excitable membranes. *Ann. Rev. Pharmacol. Toxicol.* **20**, 15.

Haller, J. S. (1984). Aconites. *Bull. N.Y. Acad. Med.* **60**, 888.

Hofmann, A. (1972). Ergot—a rich source of pharmacologically active substances. In: *Plants in the Development of Modern Medicine* (ed. T. Swain), p. 235. Harvard University Press.

Holmstedt, B. (1972). The ordeal bean of Old Calabar. In: *Plants in the Development of Modern Medicine* (ed. T. Swain), p. 303. Harvard University Press.

Lampe, K. F. (1979). Toxic fungi. *Ann. Rev. Pharmacol. Toxicol.* **19**, 85.

Matossian, M. K. (1983). The time of the Great Fear. *The Sciences,* Feb./Mar., 38.

Narahashi, T. and Wu, C. H. (1988). Mechanism of action of novel marine neurotoxins on ion channels. *Ann. Rev. Pharmacol. Toxicol.* **28**, 141.

Odell, G. V. and Ownby, C. L. (eds.) (1989). *Natural Toxins: Characterization, Pharmacology, and Therapeutics*, Proceedings of the 9th World Congress. Pergamon.

Prince, R. C. (1988). Tetrodotoxin. *Trends Pharmacol. Sci.* **13**, 26.

Rando, T., Stricharz, G., and Wang, G. K. (1987). An integrated view of the molecular toxicology of sodium channel grating in excitable cells. *Ann. Rev. Neurosci.* **10**, 237.

Schoental, R. S. (1981). Mycotoxins and foetal abnormalities. *Int. J. Environ. Sci.* **17**, 25.

Schoental, R. S. (1984). Mycotoxins and the Bible. *Perspect. Biol. Med.* **28**, 117.

Tabor, E. (1970). Plant poisons in Shakespeare. *Econ. Bot.* **24**, 81.

Thompson, C. J. S. (1934). *The Mystic Mandrake.* Rider.

Whittaker, V. P. (1990). The contribution of drugs and toxins to understanding cholinergic function. *Trends Pharmacol. Sci.* **11**, 8.

Magic

Arnold, W. N. (1989). Absinthe. *Sci. Am.* **258** (Jun.), 86.

Baudelaire, C. (1964). *Les Paradis Artificiels.* Editions Gallimard et Librairie Francaise.

Diaz, J. L. (1977). Ethnopharmacology of sacred psychoactive plants used by the Indians of Mexico. *Ann. Rev. Pharmacol. Toxicol.* **17**, 647.

Emboden, W. (1972). *Narcotic Plants.* Studio Vista.

Flores, F. A. and Lewis, W. H. (1978). Drinking the South American hallucinogenic ayahuasca. *Econ. Bot.* **32**, 154.

Griffin, W. J., Luanratana, O., and Watson, P. L. (1983). *J. Ethnopharmacol.* **8**, 303.

Hofmann, A. (1961). Chemical, pharmacological, and medical aspects of psychotomimetics. *J. Exp. Med. Sci.* **5**, 31.

Hofmann, A., Ruck, C. A. P., and Wasson, R. G. (1978). *The Road to Eleusis: Unveiling the Secrets of the Mysteries.* Harcourt Brace Jovanovich.

Hofmann, A. and Schultes, R. E. (1979). *Plants of the Gods.* Alfred Van der Mark Editions.

Huxley, A. (1968). *The Doors of Perception.* Chatto & Windus.

King, M. M. (1987). Coca Cola. *Pharm. Hist.* **29**, 85.

Lemberger, L. (1980). Potential therapeutic usefulness of marijuana. *Ann. Rev. Pharmacol. Toxicol.* **20**, 151.

Martin, R. T. (1970). Role of coca in the history, religion, and medicine of South American Indians. *Econ. Bot.* **24**, 422.

Max, B. (1990). Absinthe. *Trends Pharmacol. Sci.* **11**, 58.

Mechoulam, R. (1976). Cannabis. *La Recherche* **7**, 1018.

Russell, J. B. (1980). *A History of Witchcraft.* Thames & Hudson.

Schultes, R. E. (1969). Hallucinogens of plant origin. *Science* **163**, 245.

Spruce, R. (1908). *Notes of a Botanist on the Amazon and Andes.* Macmillan (reprinted by Johnson Reprint, 1970).

Wasson, R. G. (1968). *Soma: Divine Mushroom of Mortality.* Harcourt, Brace, and World Inc.

Medicine

Abraham, E. P., Chain, E., Fletcher, C. M., Florey, H. W., Gardner, A. D., Heatley, N. G., and Jennings, M. A. (1941). Further observations on penicillin, *Lancet* **177** (Aug.).

Anderson, F. J. (1977). *An Illustrated History of Herbals.* Columbia University Press.

Bibliography

Arber, A. (1986). *Herbals: Their Origin and Evolution* (2nd edn). Cambridge University Press.

Aronson, J. K. (1985). *An Account of the Foxglove and its Medical Uses, 1785–1985*. Oxford University Press.

Aronson, J. K. (1987). The discovery of the foxglove as a therapeutic agent. *Chem. Brit.* **23**, 33.

Berry, I. M. (1984). Feverfew faces the future. *Pharmaceutical J.* 611.

Bruce-Chwatt, L. J. and de Zulueta, J. (1980). *The Rise and Fall of Malaria in Europe*. Oxford University Press.

Bryan, C. P. (1930). *The Papyrus Ebers* (trans. from German). Bles.

Culpeper, N. (1653). *The Complete Herbal*. ICI (new edition including the *English Physician*, 1953).

Eatough, G. (1984). *Fracastoro's 'Syphilis'*. Francis Cairns.

Elvin-Lewis, M. P. F. and Lewis, W. H. (1977). *Medical Botany*. Wiley-Interscience.

Friedman, M. J. and Trager, W. (1981). The biochemistry of resistance to malaria. *Sci. Am.* **244** (Mar.), 113.

Fulder, S. (1977). Ginseng: Useless root or subtle medicine. *New Sci.* **73**, 138.

Gerard, J. (1633). *The Herbal, or General History of Plants*. Dover (1975).

Grieve, M. (1990). *A Modern Herbal*. Penguin.

Gunther, R. T. (1959). *The Greek Herbal of Dioscorides* (trans. J. Goodyer). Hafner.

Henderson, G. and McFadzean, I. (1985). Opioids—a review of recent developments. *Chem. Brit.* **21**, 1094.

Iverson, S. (1988). The chemistry of dementia. *Chem. Brit.* **24**, 338.

Jones, H., Keith, A. L., and Waddell, T. G. (1980). Legendary chemical aphrodisiacs. *J. Chem. Educ.* **57**, 341.

Krieg, M. (1965). *Green Medicine*. Harrap.

LaFond, R. E. (ed.) (1988). *Cancer: The Outlaw Cell* (2nd edn). American Chemical Society.

Leung, A. Y. (1985). *Chinese Herbal Remedies*. Wildwood House.

Macfarlane, R. G. (1979). *Howard Florey: The Making of a Great Scientist*. Oxford University Press.

Bibliography

Macfarlane, R. G. (1985). *Alexander Fleming: The Man and the Myth.* Oxford University Press.

McTavish, J. R. (1987). Aspirin in Germany. *Pharm. Hist.* **29**, 103.

Quetel, C. (1990). *History of Syphilis* (trans. J. Braddock and B. Pike). Polity Press.

Quian, S.-Z. and Wang, Z.-G. (1984). Gossypol: A potential anti-fertility agent for males. *Ann. Rev. Pharmacol. Toxicol.* **24**, 329.

Rohde, E. S. (1922). *The Old English Herbals.* Longmans, Green, & Co.

Sneader, W. (1986). *Drug Discovery: The Evolution of Modern Medicines.* Wiley.

Snyder, S. (1986). *Drugs and the Brain.* W. H. Freeman.

Stockwell, C. (1989). *Nature's Pharmacy.* Arrow Books.

Taylor, N. (1966). *Plant Drugs that Changed the World.* George Allen & Unwin.

Traynor, J. (1984). Schizophrenia: Chemistry of the split mind. *Chem. Brit.* **20**, 798.

Weissman, G. (1991). Aspirin. *Sci. Am.* **264** (Jan.), 58.

Index of scientific names

Subject index